This 50-minute DVD will introduce you to the basics of hooping
and give step-by-step instructions for some of the moves in the book.

You'll also get great warm-up exercises, workouts, and hoopdance routines.

Have fun!

HOOPING

A REVOLUTIONARY FITNESS PROGRAM

by
Christabel Zamor
with Ariane Conrad

WORKMAN PUBLISHING • NEW YORK

Library of Congress Cataloging-in-Publication Data
Zamor, Christabel.
Hooping : a revolutionary fitness program to get fit, feel sexy and have fun /
by Christabel Zamor with Ariane Conrad.
      p. cm.
Includes bibliographical references and index.
ISBN 978-0-7611-5241-5 (alk. paper)
1. Hoop exercises. 2. Exercise. I. Conrad, Ariane. II. Title.
GV490.Z36 2009
613.7'1—dc22   2008052806

WORKMAN PUBLISHING COMPANY, INC.
225 Varick Street
New York, NY 10014-4381
www.workman.com

Design by Netta Rabin
Art Direction by Janet Vicario

Disclaimer:
Because fitness and dance exercises may be physically demanding and strenuous, please consult your physician before beginning this program. Neither Workman nor HoopGirl will be liable for any complications, injuries, loss or other medical problems arising from or in connection with using this book.

Printed in the United States of America
First printing April 2009
10 9 8 7 6 5 4 3 2 1

Additional photo credits: **Bridgeman Art:** p. 18 (top, second from left); **Contact Press:** David Burnett p. 11; **Katherine Copenhaver:** p. 12; **Christopher Donald:** p. 14; **John Fenger:** pp. 114, 155; **Jenny Frederiken:** p. 98; **Getty Images:** Timothy A. Clary/AFP p. 19 (bottom, second from right), Scott Gries p. 18 (bottom, far left), Ben Martin/Time Life Pictures p. 19 (top, far right); **Sheri Giblin:** pp. 117, 133, 135, 205; **Warren Heaton/ The Hooping Life:** p. 18 (bottom, second from left); **Laurie Hobbs:** p. 156: **HoopPath:** Ann Humphreys p. 18 (bottom, third from left); **Eric Larson:** p. 52; **Manny Minjarez:** pp. 54, 100, 103, 174; **Britt Nemeth:** p. 106; **Shane Owens:** p. 154 (left and right); **Photo Researchers:** Roger Harris p. 34 (top); **Photofest:** p. 19 (bottom, far right); **Andy Pischalnikoff:** p. 128; **Pixie Vision Productions:** pp. xiv, vii (top left), 5, 19 (bottom, third from right), 34 (bottom), 107, 132; **RevellRay.com:** p. 32; **Patrick Roddie:** pp. viii (bottom left), xi, 31, 80, 188, 203; **Scott K Photography:** pp. 17 (left), 177; **Lori Weber:** pp. vi (top right), viii (top right), 17 (right), 102, 104, 158, 170; **Cully Wright:** p. 78; **Chi Young:** p. xii

This book is dedicated to you!
May you be filled with light, bliss, and joy while you whirl.
May all of your wildest dreams come true!

Acknowledgments

I'd like to start by thanking my parents, Athena and Jean-Claude, who supported me every step of the way toward hooperdom, even though they thought I was nuts at first. And without my loving husband, Kramer, none of it would have been possible. I'd also like to thank my Creator: I feel blessed with the gift of being alive.

Thanks to Amy, my superstar agent! Also to Netta and Anne at Workman, whose creative vision made this book a beautiful reality. And to Ruth, my editor, who jumped right into her own hoop to figure out what I was talking about. Her awareness of the "big picture" helped take a vast body of knowledge and distill it to its most vital components. Thank you to Scott, who took the pictures; to Shakti Activewear, which provided the wardrobe; and to all the gorgeous shining women who starred in the instructional images and the DVD: Natasha, JennaLuna, Dawn, and Ariane!

I also want to thank the other amazing women at HoopGirl, whose brilliance, passion, and hard work have made the HoopGirl educational program possible: Elaine, Andreanne, Annie, Candice, Satise, Julie, Nanette, Jess, Claudia, Ember, Susan, and Jenny. I gratefully acknowledge my hooping heroes—Anah, Rayna, Diana, Baxter and Ann, Beth, Rich, Spiral and Sharna. Your inspiring work in the field of hooping has expanded my imagination!

Finally, I am so grateful to the tens of thousands of customers, students, and fans who have sustained HoopGirl. Your interest and desire to learn more made this book possible.   —C.Z.

I am especially grateful to Caroline Paul and Antonella Moroni for their patient ears and wise advice, to Philo Hagen and Michael "Kahunahula" Henninger for holding the hooping spirit, to the Allstars and the SF Writers Grotto for their support, and to the marvelous Ruth Sullivan at Workman, who kept me smiling through rewrites and revisions.   —A.C.

Contents

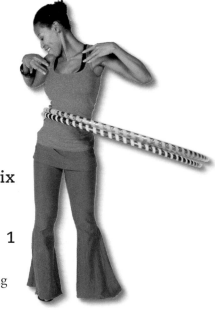

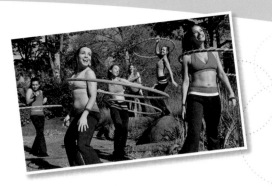

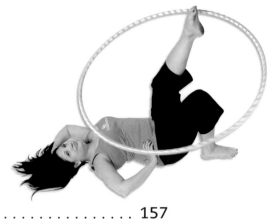

Introduction

THE STORY BEHIND HOOPGIRL

Hooping is my passion and my life's work. When people who have never seen contemporary hooping hear this, they look at me with amazement and disbelief. *You mean you stand there with a Hula Hoop® circling your waist for hours? Doesn't it get boring?* I laugh and explain that the hoop travels around my hands, upper arms, shoulders, chest, thighs, feet, both on-body and off-body. I tell them about tosses, breaks, and leaps. Hooping engages every part of my body. Beyond that, it connects me to my soul.

1950s hula-hooping has evolved into *hoopdancing,* a form of total-body fitness that sculpts abdominals, builds muscle, improves cardiovascular health, heightens endurance, and creates a lean, toned body. You don't have to be a "dancer" for hoopdancing—the hoop's rhythmic bump on your body educates your body to move with the beat. All you have to do is interact with the hoop and respond to it.

Upon discovering the hoop for myself—a story I'll share next—and recognizing the fantastic physical, emotional, and spiritual benefits, I created a company and a curriculum so I could spread the joy of hooping. This book and DVD are the result of my near-decade of learning, teaching, and sharing.

In the book I lay out the basic HoopGirl Workout Program and philosophy. You'll learn over fifty HoopGirl moves—plus combinations—that engage your core, arms, and legs, providing a total body workout. You'll meet people who tell you how hoopdancing has transformed them in ways that go way beyond physical fitness. You'll hear from doctors and other health experts who recommend hooping for healing and preventing a number of common ailments, from back pain and circulation problems to bone loss and stress. And because it's useful to learn exercise by watching, the book comes with a DVD that demonstrates basic hoop moves and provides a 50-minute workout.

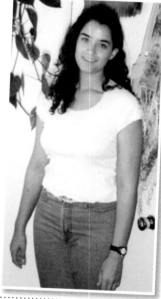

Before . . .

The Genesis of HoopGirl

I did not hoop as a child. Ever. When I picked up my first hoop, I was twenty-seven years old and working on a doctoral degree in cultural anthropology. I was overweight, awkward, and introverted. I hid my body in dark, baggy clothes. I compulsively smoked cigarettes every time I set foot outdoors. And I had a lot of pain with my periods that turned out to be a disease called endometriosis. The medications I took for it decreased my sex drive and made me question my femininity and sex appeal. For multiple reasons, I wasn't "in my body" much of the time.

Then one day at a music festival I noticed people playing with hoops. They made it look effortless and fun. Someone tossed me one so I could give it a whirl. For about twenty minutes I attempted to get the thing spinning around my waist. It fell down. It knocked against my hipbones. It fell again, and again and again. The hoopers gave me some pointers and encouraged me, smiling sympathetically, but I was embarrassed. I fled.

Still, something about the sensation of the hoop rolling over my pelvis, for even just one revolution, had me hooked. I got myself a hoop and headed to a park to practice alone, soon getting the hang of spinning it around my waist. It wasn't long before my weekly practice sessions weren't enough. Utterly consumed, I spent every free moment hooping, even in my tiny living space. It was the most fun I'd had in ages.

The first effect I noticed was that I lost the urge to smoke. If I ever did have a craving, I'd pick up my intoxicating hoop instead of a cigarette. It was a wonderful alternative way to release stress and unwind. My body began changing in a matter of weeks, too. I was more toned and my jeans got looser. Over the next six months, my unwanted extra fat just disappeared and was replaced by gorgeous muscle. I started wearing more revealing clothes so my bare skin could touch and grip the hoop . . . and I felt fantastic in them.

I also noticed that I was thinking differently. I felt a deep sense of joyfulness that persisted for longer and longer periods of time. Hooping was loosening me up. I smiled and laughed every day and took myself less seriously. I found myself looking for things to admire in the people around me instead of things to criticize. I started appreciating my life.

Above all, the undulations brought my awareness back into my body, specifically to the region of my pelvic area. The soothing gyrations reminded the anthropologist in me of other cultures' sacred ritual dances for menstruation and childbirth. I would still need to have surgeries on my ovaries for the endometriosis, but once I recovered from the procedures, my hoop helped me heal.

. . . and after.

I also realized that up until this point I had relied on others to make me feel feminine. Gradually, with the help of my hoop, I came to understand that my femininity originated from within. Once I connected with that inner power, I felt exuberant, delightful, and sassy—I felt *sexy*. This sensation of sexy had nothing to do with *sex,* per se; it was a sense of self-love, inner ease, and confidence. With the hoop as my partner, I learned to develop these qualities, independent of anyone else.

In a culture where we spend so much time sitting at desks and are discouraged from moving our hips (at least in public), hooping was a profound awakening for me. I knew I had to share my discoveries, especially with other women. I began holding a weekly hoop event and shared hooping with everyone I knew. Soon, phone calls and e-mails were pouring in from people seeking hoops, classes, and guidance and asking if I was "the hoop girl." That was the beginning of my company, HoopGirl, which has exploded into an empire of group classes, instructional DVDs, performances, and teacher certification programs. My HoopGirl Workout was approved by the American Aerobics and Fitness Association (AAFA) and has been adopted by health clubs such as Crunch and Curves so is now available in gyms nationwide.

The HoopGirl company motto is "Get Fit, Feel Sexy, Have Fun." My courses provide challenging, multilevel workouts that improve strength, balance, coordination, flexibility, and resilience. Classes take place in circles with freeform movement, as opposed to static lines facing the mirror. There is always time for students to set an intention (such as "to release this week's stress" or "to reawaken my feminine side"), warm up, learn moves, focus on a specific part of the body, play games, perform in a jam circle, and cool down. I encourage laughter, pleasure, and the abandon of ecstatic dance. It is much more than a fitness class—it is an *experience* that builds connection, confidence, and friendships. For readers of this book, you may want to keep a hooping journal to record your experiences and insights. Look back at your successes, review practice sessions, and stay positive.

I constantly witness students transforming themselves. Many arrive at class with a hangdog look, confessing that they could never hoop as a kid, their body language clearly indicating they expect to fail again. It's my great honor to show them how to achieve orbit, and to see the delight in their flushed faces at the end of our first class together. I've watched countless women swap their oversize T-shirts and sweatpants for body-hugging cropped tops and shorts as their confidence in their bodies skyrockets. I love nurturing liberation, flamboyance, and assertiveness in my students. Most of all, I adore laughing with them and learning from them.

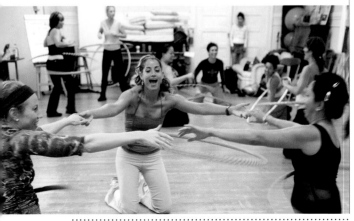

Connecting during class

What to Expect from Hooping

While hooping is a phenomenal workout, it can be far more than that. It's a state of mind, a lifestyle, and a way of interacting, becoming, and being. Some of the advantages of regular hooping include:

FOR THE BODY

Improves core strength

Improves motor skills

Heightens stamina and energy

Improves balance

Sculpts abdominals, arms, thighs, and buns

Builds hand-eye coordination

Enhances articulation of joints

Delivers a cardio-aerobic workout

Enhances somatic and kinesthetic intelligence

Unwinds and realigns the spine

Strengthens neurological pathways

Accelerates fat burning and weight loss

Strengthens back muscles

Boosts libido!

Improves flexibility and dexterity

Improves posture and alignment

Deepens breath

Develops a sense of rhythm

FOR THE MIND AND SPIRIT

Promotes laughter

Encourages pleasurable sensations

Boosts self-esteem and confidence

Quiets/focuses the mind

Helps overcome shyness

Establishes boundaries around the body

Creates a sense of flow

Encourages creativity and imagination

Relieves stress

Develops trust in one's body

Restores the body-mind-spirit connection

Imparts a sense of freedom

Develops a "Yes I Can!" attitude

Centers and calms the emotions

Promotes cooperation and community

Establishes connectedness to the body

Helps one reclaim a sense of power

Promotes happiness and well-being

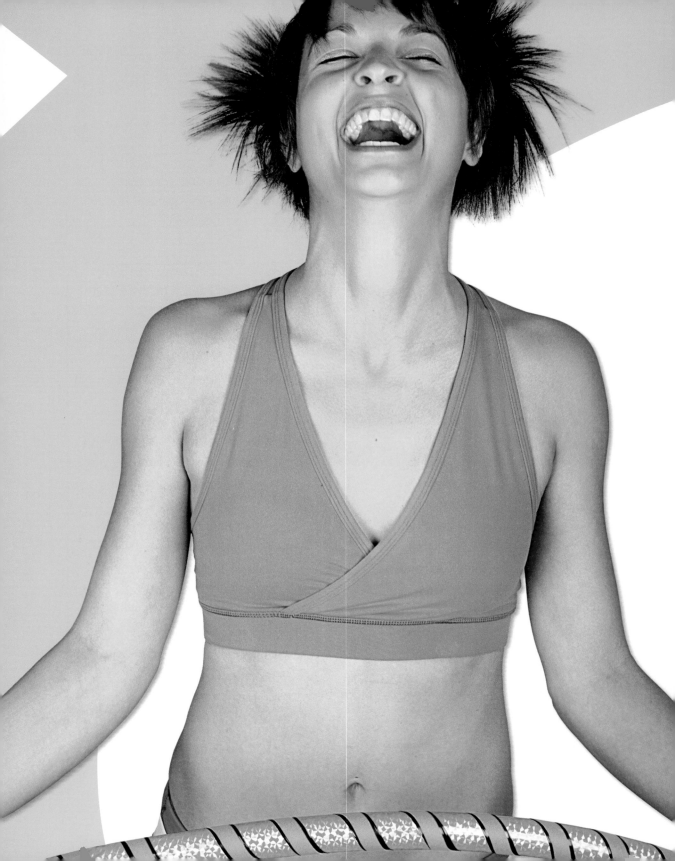

Fitness as Fun

LIMBER UP YOUR
MUSCLES & YOUR MIND

Close your eyes for a minute and use all five senses to scoop up memories from when you were a kid. Maybe you remember running squealing through the sprinkler, toes squishing the slick grass . . . Yelling sound effects like POW! and VROOM! while playing pretend . . . Or improvising a rhythm section with pots and wooden spoons. Sitting still was *boring,* so you bounced, wriggled, and twirled nonstop. You felt carefree and invincible, and the whole world was yours to discover. Magic in the smallest things took your breath away.

You're about to feel like that again. Welcome to hooping! The secret to the raging popularity of hooping as exercise is simple: It's *fun.* In fact, it's so much fun that once you start, you won't be able to put your hoop down.

The sheer silliness of hooping stands in stark contrast to the regimented routines of mainstream fitness. Lots of traditional exercise devotees still cling to Jane Fonda's 1980s mantra of "no pain, no gain" and "feel the burn," even if they've traded her aerobic routines for elliptical trainers, weights, or kickboxing classes. Most people expect and accept physical discomfort (and mental monotony) from exercise. They "whip" their bodies into shape and push past pain in their muscles and joints. And usually they're *paying* for the experience, to the tune of $50 to $100 per month.

The biggest problem with other fitness regimes is that people don't stick with them. They may start out with the best intentions, but usually lose interest, get bored, or won't follow through. At the core of the HoopGirl Workout is the Pleasure Principle, which means that *play* replaces the *work* in workout because it feels so good. Suddenly, instead of

"With my 40- to 50-hour workweek, the last thing I want to do is spend more of my precious time away from my family at a gym. Hooping gives a great workout, plus my kids can hoop with me or play nearby."

—Jodie, 40

dreading the boring reps and stale air of the gym, you'll find you can hardly wait to give your hoop another spin.

As one HoopGirl student put it: "I hate the gym. The machines and the people make me feel insecure—I just want to get out of there as soon as possible. But with my hoop I have so much fun, I can keep going for hours on end!" The hoop brings a childlike sense of play back into physical movement, the kind of giddy, giggly joy you probably haven't felt since you were a kid.

My beginners' classes are always filled with whooping, hollering, and laughter—lots and lots of laughter. And it's coming from the fifty-somethings as much as from the twenty- and thirty-year-olds! The hoop gives everyone permission to be raucous, like they've been let out for recess. *Wheee! Look at me! I'm doing it! I'm doing it!* fills the room once the hoops get going. Within the first half hour, most students start to pant and glisten, completely surprised by how much energy it takes to keep the hoop in motion. Their eyes get wider. Shoulders and hips get flirty. Someone pulls a Travolta *Saturday Night Fever* move, one dramatic finger pointing. Another starts voguing.

The Pleasure Principle means you can let yourself go—there's no dignity to preserve here. Take risks. Be silly. Let the hoop bumping against you guide your movement,

Laughing Exercise

HERE'S A BREATHING EXERCISE ADAPTED FROM Laughter Yoga that warms up the abdominal muscles before hooping and increases the amount of oxygen in your body. As it turns out, normal inhalation fills just 75 percent of the lungs; the remaining 25 percent of space in there is filled with stale air that never gets cleared out in regular breathing! The goal here is to expel all that residual air and allow revitalizing, energizing oxygen to saturate the body. So your exhalation should go on and on and on, like the Energizer bunny.

This exercise induces laughter, but there's no sense of humor required. The physical act of belly laughter tones muscles, assists circulation, oxygenates your body, and boosts your immune system. At first, it may feel forced to laugh on cue, but studies have shown that your body doesn't know the difference between real and fake laughter, so the endorphins are released regardless, flooding your system with happy hormones. Did you know that adults laugh a paltry fifteen times per day, on average, while kids laugh about four hundred times a day? You have a lot of catching up to do!

1 Stand comfortably with your feet hip-width apart, your knees slightly bent, and inhale deeply. On the exhale, raise your arms while saying the word *"hoooo-laaaa."* Raise the pitch of your voice and extend the word. Pull your shoulders slightly back to open your heart and expand the space between your ribs. Hold your breath for a few seconds while feeling a stretch throughout your entire body.

2 Then, with hands clasped together overhead, bend forward at the waist, and with your mouth open wide let the exhalation come out as loud laughter—*ha ha ha ha!* The laugh happens after you think you've already exhaled as much as you possibly can. Repeat and keep the laughs coming!

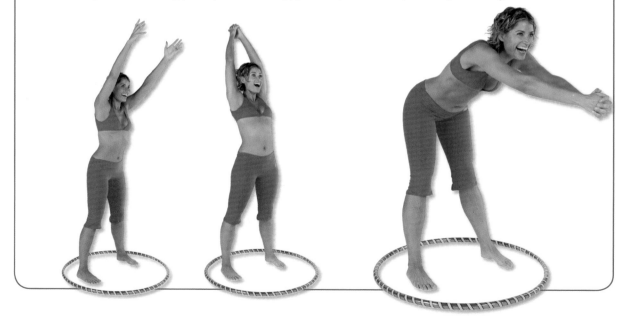

like you're playing follow the leader. Allow every joint in your body to come alive and move in ways that feel good: fingers, wrists, elbows, shoulders, knees, ankles, and above all, your hips. And if the pelvic rocking brings up some primal movements or sounds from inside you, give yourself over to them. It's all good.

Another aspect of the Pleasure Principle is to *stop if it hurts*. While you're still new to hooping, you may develop bruises on your hips. To prevent this, keep your hoop sessions short at first—even though you'll probably be tempted to go for longer. As you learn to maneuver the hoop around other contact points like your elbows, knees, and knuckles, pay attention to tender spots. If something hurts, take a break!

To be sustainable, exercise needs to entertain you and feel good. It's a no-brainer: If it delights and tickles you, you'll want more of it! In hooping classes I've watched thousands of students get hooked, and stay hooked. Hooping's fun factor captivates to the point of being *addictive*—to new students and veteran hoopers alike.

Getting in Shape

OK, you're saying. *I'll have fun. I'll giggle and wriggle and prance like a kid. I might even channel Madonna or Xena.*

But will it get me in shape? According to thousands of HoopGirl students and tens of thousands of hoopers worldwide, the answer is a resounding yes! Their physical transformations include smaller waistlines, tightened abs, defined arms, pounds lost, and rejuvenated complexions. But don't take it from me.

Dr. Jan Schroeder is a big deal in the world of exercise science. As a professor of kinesiology, she's a researcher and a lead consultant to IDEA, the largest fitness association in the country. And she's a hooper herself! Dr. Schroeder is conducting clinical studies at California State University to prove that regular hooping (one hour twice a week) improves cardiorespiratory endurance, flexibility, balance, and muscular endurance.

She notes that hooping impacts *every* muscle in the core, including the small muscles that can be difficult to reach with most forms of exercise. "Plus," she adds, "once I learned that the hoop doesn't just circle the core, but the upper torso, arms, and legs, it opened up the terrain of whole-body fitness."

One of the main reasons she favors hooping is that it moves your body in multiple directions. Our bodies are *engineered* for a range of activities: Think of early humans reaching to pluck berries, running from a predator, climbing trees to pick fruit, bending to collect wood, and digging for roots. "Hooping has an irregular loading pattern," says Schroeder, "while activities like running, walking, cycling, or fitness machines have a very linear, continuous loading pattern on the body. But that's not natural. In everyday life, the body has to constantly adjust, compensate, reach, and move in new and different directions." Hooping mimics this kind of impulsive motion—and better prepares the body for it.

With traditional exercises and machines (like stair-climbers and treadmills) it doesn't take long before your body goes on autopilot, working the same old muscles with fewer and fewer results. By contrast, the very unpredictability of hooping—its zaniness!—is what makes it such an outstanding workout.

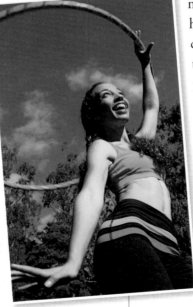

You didn't think hooping made its way onto so many Top Ten Ways to Get Fit lists, or is now offered at thousands of gyms just because it's FUN, did you? Not only is hooping a great *aerobic workout,* it also *builds strength* and *increases flexibility*—the three types of activities that fitness experts say are necessary for a full-body workout.

Easing Into It: Stretching

As with any form of exercise, if you stretch first, your body will thank you. The following HoopGirl warm-up moves loosen muscles, raise your heart rate, and increase the flow of blood and oxygen throughout your body. They also set the spunky, sassy mood for hoopdance.

You don't have to do all these exercises every time, but always do at least five minutes of stretching before any hoop session. If you're short on time, choose specific warm-ups to prepare the muscles and joints you know you'll be using. Breathe deeply. As a general rule, remember to *ex*hale with the *ex*ertion. Practice flexing your smile along with your body.

Use these same stretches after hooping to cool down. Stretching after a workout increases your flexibility, helps to remove lactic acid from your muscles, and minimizes soreness.

QUAD STRETCH   target zone ▶ LEGS

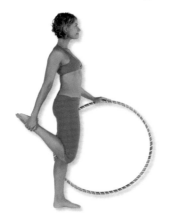

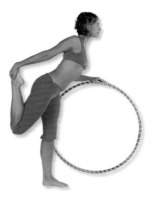

1 Stand with your feet shoulder-width apart. Place the hoop at your left side, and rest your left hand on it. Now grasp your right ankle with your right hand, lifting it toward your buttocks. (If you can't do this stretch easily, use a yoga strap to help reach your ankle.)

2 Keep your back straight and keep your bent knee from drifting ahead of your standing leg. Deepen the stretch by leaning forward and pulling your heel closer to your bun. Hold to the count of 3. Then switch sides.

NECK ROLLS   target zone ▶ NECK

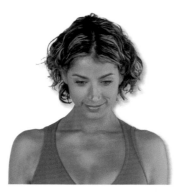

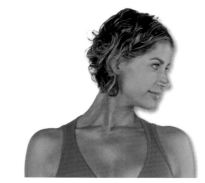

1 Keeping your shoulders down and relaxed, tilt your head forward so your chin drops slightly toward your chest. Make a complete circle with your neck, inhaling as you roll your head up to the right and exhaling as you roll down and around to the left.

2 Be careful not to tilt your head back. To protect the delicate vertebrae at your neck, imagine you're tracing a circle with the tip of your nose on a window right in front of you. Do five full circles in one direction then reverse direction for five more.

SPINAL TWIST target zone ▶ ABS–BACK

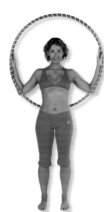 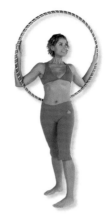

1 Stand with your feet shoulder-width apart, holding the hoop behind you so that the bottom is at the small of your back and the top frames your head. Breathing deeply and keeping your lower body stationary, twist just your upper torso to the right. Pause.

2 Then twist to the left until you feel a gentle, satisfying stretch. Keep your head up and the hoop on a flat vertical plane against your back. Breathe steadily as you twist four more times to each side.

TORSO DIPS target zone ▶ HIPS–BACK–LEGS

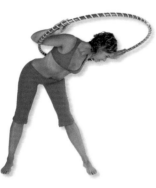 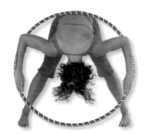

1 Stand holding the hoop behind your back (as for Spinal Twist, above) and inhale. Slowly exhale as you bend diagonally forward from the hips so the top of the hoop swings down toward your left foot. (Your hoop may graze the floor—this is fine.) Feel the gentle stretch in your left hamstring and along your right side.

2 Still bending forward, sweep the hoop along the space between your legs to your right foot, feeling the opposite stretch. Inhale as you rise slowly until you are standing with the hoop behind your back. Imagine you're a windmill doing slow and steady revolutions in the breeze. Repeat four times, then reverse direction.

HIP SWAYS   target zone ▶ HIPS–ABS–BACK

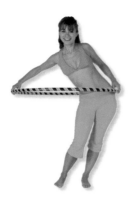

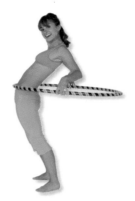

1 Hold the hoop suspended at waist level, your feet shoulder-width apart. In slow, wide movements, swing your hips to the left and then swing them to the right while holding the hoop still. Breathe. Try to touch the inside of the hoop with your hips. Repeat ten times.

2 Now swing your hips to the front and to the back, ten times in each direction. This is the same movement you do to keep the hoop in its basic orbit so it's good to impress it on your muscular memory. Keep your shoulders back and down and your head up.

LIFT + CROUCH   target zone ▶ LEGS–ARMS

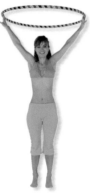

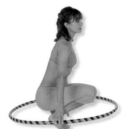

1 Stand holding the hoop around you (as in Hip Sways, above). As you exhale, lift the hoop up, extending your arms fully so the hoop is above your head like a halo. Rise up onto your tiptoes to get an extra stretch in your calves.

2 Then bring the hoop back down to hip level, inhale and squat down, dropping your buns back and down as if to sit on a chair. (If you have problems with your knees, skip this warm-up.) Keep your shoulders back and down and your back straight. Now lift and crouch as one continual movement. Repeat the move ten times.

SHOULDER SHIMMIES   target zone ▶ SHOULDERS–BACK

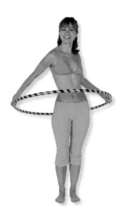

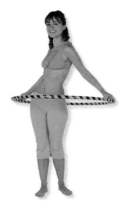

1 Stand, holding the hoop at your waist with a light, flexible grip. Push your right shoulder forward as you pull the left one backward. Now push your left shoulder forward while you pull the right one back. Keep the hoop and your lower body as still as possible. Breathe!

2 Imagine that you have maracas in your shoulders as you begin to speed up the alternating forward and back movement. Make the motion contained, percussive, and continuous. Keep shimmying until you feel tingly and warm, about one minute.

PUSH-OUTS   target zone ▶ ARMS–LEGS

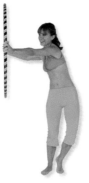

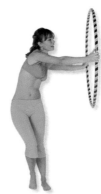

1 Begin a step-touch with your feet, where you step to the right side with the right foot and bring the left to touch it, then step to the left side with your left foot and bring the right to touch. Let your whole body take on the rhythm. Now pick up the hoop and push it out to the side—in the same direction you're stepping.

2 As you step to the right, push the hoop out to your right side. Your right arm should extend straight out to the side. Then step to the left as you push the hoop to the left. Do ten on each side.

Breathe Easy

DO YOU KNOW THE LUNGS ARE THE ONLY ORGAN of the body that we can immediately influence? Being able to control and slow your breathing is vital to hooping. It relaxes your body and calms your mind, so that no matter how hard you exert yourself, how fast and long you spin, or how high you jump, you can maintain control, balance, and grace.

Pranayama Yoga is the practice of elongating the breath to increase life force energy. Hoopers draw on this practice by consciously deepening and lengthening our inhalations and exhalations. This kind of breathing allows you to stay focused, alert, and present in your body while you take on physical challenges. Inspirations—in the literal sense of breathing in—lead to true inspiration!

Sit comfortably in a chair or on the floor, with your shoulders back and down to "open" your heart. If you're unfamiliar with Prana breathing, begin your breath awareness by placing your hands on your abdomen. Inhale through your nose, filling your abdomen completely. (Feel your belly expand under your hands.) Continue to inhale, next filling your chest (expanding the rib cage), then fill the top of your lungs (so your clavicle rises). Pause for a moment, then exhale in the opposite order, releasing your breath first from the top of the lungs, then the chest, and last the abdomen. Be sure to expel all the breath from the belly (with your hands, feel your abs pull toward your spine). Pause. As you inhale, imagine you are inflating two large balloons in your belly and chest. As you exhale, imagine your lungs flat and pressed together, like vacuum-packed ziplock bags.

Repeat. This time, try putting a count to your inhalations and exhalations. Inhale to the count of 3 and exhale to the count of 3, again filling all three areas of your chest cavity. Gradually increase the length of your exhalation so that it is twice as long as your inhalation. In other words, if you inhale to a count of 3, exhale to a count of 6 or whatever number is comfortable for you. After a few rounds of this, return your breath to normal. Pause and notice how your body feels.

Limber Up Your Mind

It's often a student's mind that gets in the way of mastering a physical challenge. Let go of any experiences you may have had with hooping in the past and create a can-do attitude. Hooping is fun, and you, too, can master it. Yes, you can!

Take your cue from top athletes, who use visualization to land high scores and gold medals. Figure skaters imagine their bodies elevated for the full third turn of a triple lutz. Tennis stars visualize their serves swerving into an ace. Runners see themselves flying across the finish line in record-breaking time. There's a reason why athletes do this: It works!

Now visualize yourself inside a hoop's orbit: Your hips swing rhythmically. Your feet push into the floor like pylons while your spine swerves gracefully. Your torso moves easily to greet the hoop every time you feel the hoop press against you. Your arms flow like quicksilver. Your powerhouse core fuels a dynamic dance. Exhilaration and perspiration make your skin glow. The pulsing of the hoop quiets your thoughts; you breathe deep from your belly and smile from the center of your being.

And if your hoop does clatter to the floor the first few times—or even the tenth or twentieth time—focus on feeling *fascination* rather than frustration. Become intrigued by the challenge of mastering a new skill. Commit to your success. And remember to be compassionate and patient with your body. Babies don't stand up and walk immediately—they take time to find their balance and strength.

During my first attempt at hooping, I flailed around for twenty minutes as the hoop fell again and again! Yet that one moment when the hoop encircled me before falling was so exhilarating, I vowed to feel it again. Remember how many times you fell off your first bike only to climb back in the saddle? That's how this is. The rush of *getting* it—of actually doing it, even for a second—will power your persistence.

Focus first on getting that single revolution of the hoop around your body. Savor the success and then build on it. Take even the smallest moments of hooping ease as signs that *yes you can do it*. You are well on your way to achieving orbit!

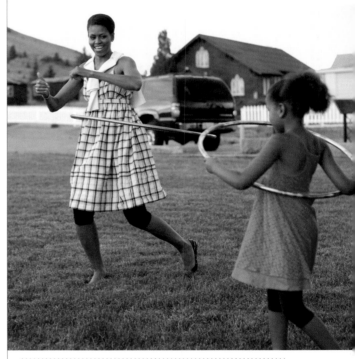

First Lady Michelle Obama and daughter Sasha give the hoop a whirl

Out of Hiding Into the Circle

I REMEMBER BEING AT RAVES WHERE I'D SEE skinny girls dancing in hoops and I'd think: I could never do what they did. I'm apple-shaped, you know? But I bought myself a hoop anyway because I knew it would be good for weight loss. Once it arrived, it sat in the corner for months. It called out to me, but I was too embarrassed to try it with my roommates around.

In the meantime I was doing everything I could to bring myself under 200 pounds. I went to the gym five days a week and did a lot of aerobic stuff like the treadmill and the elliptical trainer. I severely restricted my diet, to the point where I was eating tiny portions of rabbit food every day, and that was it. Salads, salads, and more salads.

Finally one day when there was no one around to watch, I tried out my hoop. I was amazed at how good it felt! It didn't feel like exercise, it was just fun. And I quickly found I could do things I never imagined possible. I could actually feel strength, stamina, and agility in the body I'd spent so much time hating and hiding. After a while I got less self-conscious and took

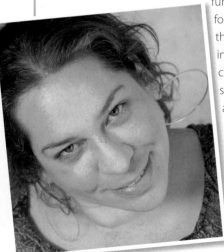

some classes and sometimes went to local meet-ups with other hoopers. Once I was inside my hoop I felt kind of like no one was watching me anyway—it was like the hoop was the star, not me.

Still concerned about my weight and health, I went to doctors, dieticians, and personal trainers. I took various tests for my metabolism, and my personal trainers made me wear an armband that recorded my body heat in order to see how many calories I was burning. I had to wear it all the time for a week straight, even when I was asleep—everywhere except in the shower.

The results were pretty mind-blowing to my personal trainer and my doctor. During Christabel's hoop class I was burning ten calories a minute, or six hundred calories an hour. The elliptical trainer had met its match!

In the end, the doctors determined that my metabolism had slowed down so dramatically to compensate for my starvation diet that I couldn't lose any weight. So I started eating normally again—you have no idea what a relief and a joy that has been—and I kept hooping.

Now I'm not tiny by any stretch, but I'm toned, and I eat like a regular person. And I find myself thinking: I can't be all that unattractive—I can do some pretty dope moves! And above all, I've developed discipline and focus that parallels my physical transformation. That makes me proud and confident.

Name: Holly
Occupation: Software Piracy Investigator

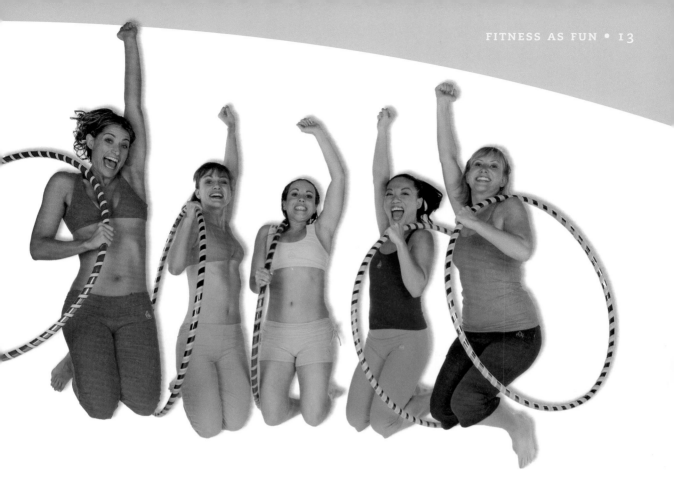

Yes I Can! Journal Exercise

GIVE YOUR ATTITUDE A WORKOUT BEFORE GIVING THE HOOP A WHIRL.

If you find your mind doubting your ability to achieve orbit within the hoop, this writing exercise can pump up your confidence. Reflect for a moment and remember the last time you were asked to do something you'd never done before, when, despite your doubts in your own ability, you met the challenge. How did your achievement make you feel? What kinds of sensations flooded your body and your mind? Where in your body did you feel them specifically?

Write a few sentences in your hooping journal (see page xii) about each stage in the process: the doubt(s), the attempt(s), the success(es), the feeling(s), and the learning(s). Describe it as though you're sharing the story of your proud accomplishment with a close friend, using visual details and metaphors so she really gets it.

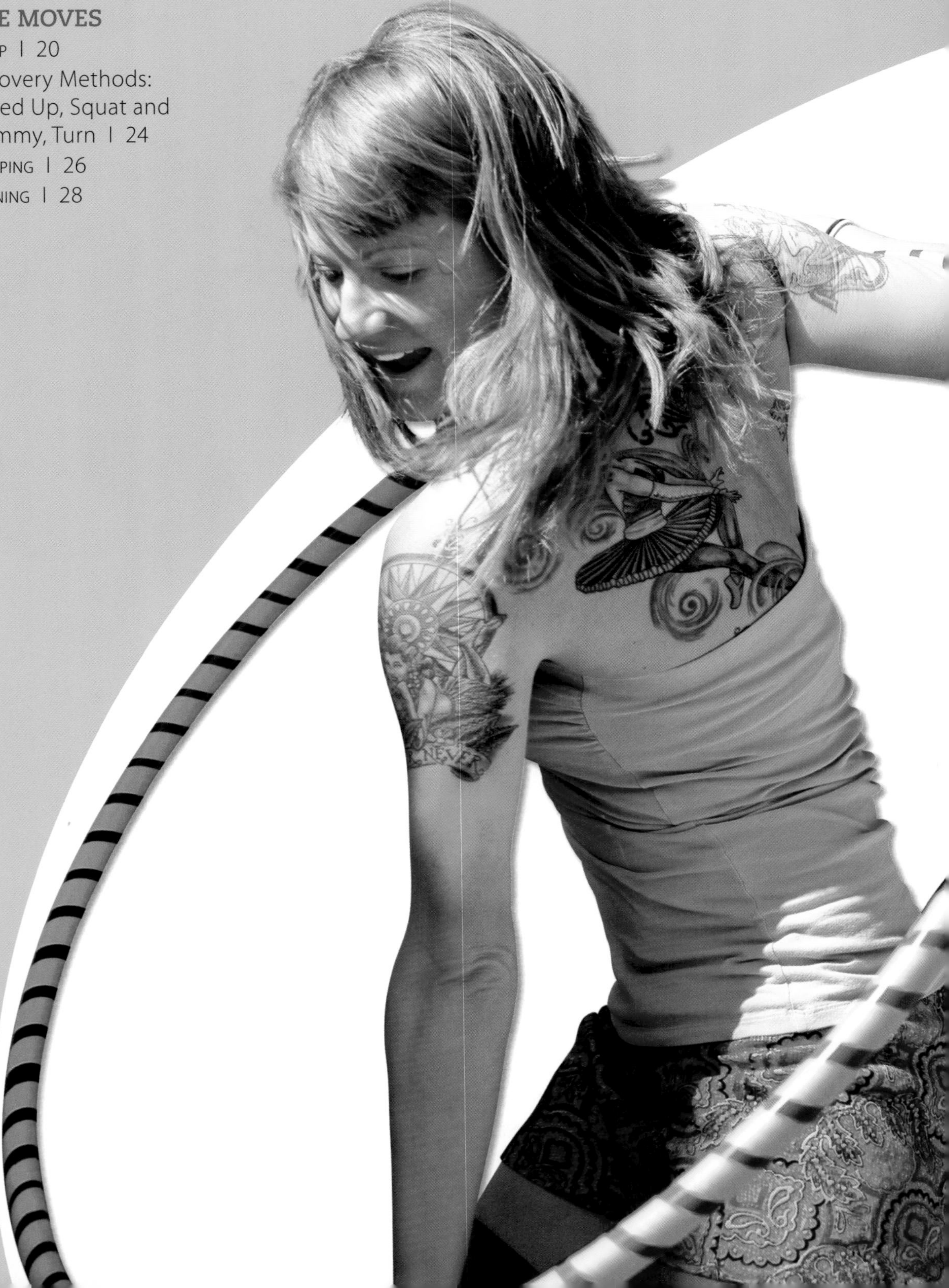

The Evolution of Revolution

HOOPING COMES FULL CIRCLE

I f you can walk, you can hoop! It doesn't matter how old you are, or how out of shape. Your measurements don't matter either: Goddess-size women can use proportionate hoops to rock their world. That's because hoops have evolved; they're now made to fit adult bodies and are covered with fabric tapes that help them adhere to your body.

And hoopers are everywhere. It doesn't matter where you live—people are hooping on blacktops and roofs, in gyms and on suburban lawns, in the snow and on the beach. Because you can do it anywhere, there's no expensive gym membership involved. It's low-tech! No cables, chrome, or sharp edges. No assembly required. All you need is hips—and a hoop of your own. (See page 16 for information on buying a hoop.)

Hooping has grown up. The playground pastime and romper room activity has transformed into *hoopdance,* a sweat-drenching, accredited form of exercise for the total body. Today there are tens of thousands of hoopers worldwide, using online social networks (like YouTube and Facebook) to seek advice, share tricks and videos, and connect . . . so that they can meet up in person, 2.0 style, to hoop, sweat, and laugh together. The revolution is here!

The Basics

The one and only thing you need to join in the fun is . . . a hoop.

I'm not talking about a hoop from the toy store. Those are made for children's bodies, and are too small and light for most adults. I'm talking about an adult-size hoop, one with a larger diameter and made of thicker tubing. When it's standing on the ground in front of you, your hoop should come up to a few inches above your belly button. As a general rule of thumb: The bigger you are, the bigger the hoop should be.

Larger hoops rotate more slowly, which makes them easier to control and simpler to learn on. I think of them as training wheels. Because they are made of heavier tubing, they provide greater resistance, which makes them good for strength

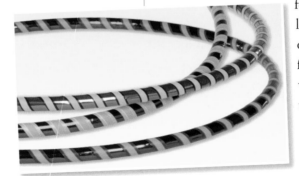

"Being a hooper in Tokyo has allowed me to create a beautiful personal space in a city that makes it tough to find your own space. Now I shine and stand out, in a city of over thirteen million people!"
—Deanne, 32

training (even at a pound and a half) and brings you to a sweat faster. There are also lighter-weight adult-diameter hoops that zip around your body in much less time. Their speed makes learning core moves challenging. Hoopdancers often graduate to smaller hoops as they gain proficiency.

For an average price of $30, you can buy a hoop online. For hooping vendors, see the "Online Hoop Resources" in the Appendix, page 202. HoopGirl hoops are custom-crafted to be the optimal weight for fun and weight loss—about twenty-one to twenty-five ounces—and wrapped with fabric tapes that help the hoop "stick" to you.

Once you've got your hoop, you'll need a spot to spin in. For basic hooping around your waist, you need only as much space as the hoop takes up in its revolution around your body, or about a six-by-six-foot square. When you start experimenting with off-body moves, you'll need more space both horizontally around you (at least three times the diameter of the hoop), and vertically above you. For most people, this means heading outside to a park or a rooftop, or into one of the unoccupied spaces with high ceilings at your local gym.

THREADS

Obviously, wear something that allows you to move and groove in every direction. As fabrics go, cotton and stretch denim are good hoopable choices. Watch out for slippery synthetics such as rayon, polyester, or Lycra, which allow the hoop to slide off more easily. More than anything, hoops love bare skin—it's the "grippiest" surface. Sports bras or bikini tops are good for exposing your core.

As for your feet, hooping barefoot—especially outdoors, in the grass or on the beach—evokes the freedom and bliss of childhood. Try it! But if you're doing a lot of bouncing and jumping with your hoop, wear athletic shoes for support. If you're twirling and gliding indoors, you may want to try dance sneakers, which reduce friction like grease on a griddle.

Now all you need to do is turn up the volume on some good hip-grooving tunes, and you're ready to learn the fundamental move that keeps the hoop rotating around your core, PUMP. Music helps you have fun and experiment with dance! To get you started, there are sample playlists throughout the book that match the mood of the moves in each chapter.

Rocking the tube top

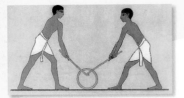

1000 BC
Egyptian children play with large hoops of dried grapevines and stiff grasses. The toy is propelled along the ground with a stick or swung around the waist.

500 BC
Greek boys play and exercise with hoops made of bronze, called a trochus, which they roll along the ground.

1400s
Healers among the Lakota Indians develop hoop dances (to them, the hoop represents the circle of life) in ceremonies for restoring balance and harmony in the world. The dancers use dozens of small, lightweight hoops made of reeds to tell stories and imitate natural forms such as eagles, butterflies, or rain.

LATE 1500s
As part of the Christian festivities before the fasting period of Lent, French girls dance inside wooden hoops, wearing floral garlands.

EARLY 1800s
Hoops achieve fad status in England. Children play with wooden hoops, using a stick called a skimmer to roll them along ("hoop bowling") or swinging them around the waist as in modern hooping.

Hoops Come Full Circle

What goes around comes around. The hoop (or some version of it) sure has, cycling in and out of popularity, but always returning. Centuries before the Wham-O corporation came along in the 1950s and popularized their Hula Hoops® made out of plastic tubing, people were playing with hoops made of flexible branches, reeds, and vines. Here's a brief look at the many places where hoops have rolled across the stage of history.

2008-2009
Hoopdance is anointed by *Time* magazine and other major national media as one of the hottest new fitness trends and is featured on MTV, *The Today Show,* and *Good Morning America,* and in the pages of *Vogue* and *Shape* magazines.

2007–2009
Celebrities such as Beyoncé, Carmen Electra, Gwyneth Paltrow, and Michelle Obama come out as hoopers. Macka Diamond releases her hit song "Hoola Hoop."

2006
Filming begins on the feature-length documentary *The Hooping Life,* which follows the lives of six icons in the modern world of hooping.

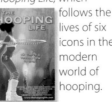

JULY 2006
Hoopdancer Anah "Hoopaliscious" Reichenbach appears on *America's Got Talent.*

2006
Jonathan Baxter develops a ground-breaking hooping curriculum of techniques that use breaks and reversals to punctuate the hoop's flow.

2005
The Scissor Sisters release the video for their hit "Filthy/Gorgeous," which features glam transvestite hoopdancer, Karis.

1940s–1950s
Hoops made of cane are used in Australian schools, where children swing hoops around their waists, knees, and arms, and perform these moves for the Queen.

1958
Richard Knerr and Arthur Melin, founders of Wham-O, manufacture a plastic hoop. Twenty-five million Hula-Hoops® are sold in the U.S. in four months! By 1959, sales hit 100 million.

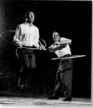

LATE 1800s
British sailors visiting the Hawaiian Islands notice parallels between the hip motions of native hula dances and the popular activity back home in England. They attach the word "hula" to "hoop."

1942
Native American hoop dancer White Cloud makes a cameo appearance in *Valley of the Sun*, starring Lucille Ball, and appears again in Gene Autry's movie *Apache Country*.

1960s
Circus performers integrate multiple hoops into their acts, particularly in Russia and China.

1990s
Jam-band The String Cheese Incident throws hoops out to its audiences, sowing the seeds for the new millennium's incarnation of hooping.

Today hoopdancers appear everywhere on stage in the glamorous worlds of fashion, music, and film. Burlesque, belly dance, hip-hop, circus acrobatics, rhythmic gymnastics, yoga, and the electronic music scene have cross-pollinated with hooping to create new fusion dance-forms. Hoops have come back around, and they're here to stay!

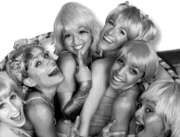

AUGUST 2003
Hoops explode onto the scene at Burning Man, the annual festival of arts and freedom in the Nevada desert.

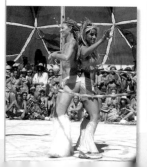

2003
The Good Vibe Hoop Tribe, an all-female hoopdance performance troupe, forms in Los Angeles, soon followed by the coed Groovehoops in New York City (2003), the HoopGirl Allstars in San Francisco, above (2006), and the Whirly Girlz in Portland, Oregon (2006).

APRIL 2003
Hooping.org, the world's first hooping publication, is launched.

2000s
Cirque du Soleil features dazzling acrobats maneuvering multiple hoops.

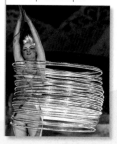

1994
The Coen Brothers' film *The Hudsucker Proxy* gives a fictional account of the invention of the hoop, aka the "extruded plastic dingus."

Pump

Use your hips to propel the hoop around the waist on the horizontal plane. Contrary to what some beginners think, it's a forward-back pelvic push-pull, rather than a circular hip motion, that propels the hoop.

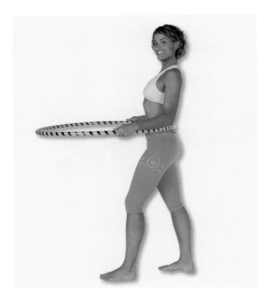

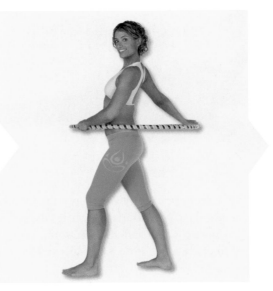

1 Stand inside the hoop with one foot slightly in front of the other and your knees slightly bent. Your feet need to be far enough apart to stabilize you during a wild ride of hip thrusting, or about one foot's length apart. Avoid widening your stance beyond that. (Spreading your legs out will not help you keep the hoop up, despite how it may feel!)

2 Hold the hoop in your hands at waist level, so it rests against the small of your back. Twist your upper torso to wind the hoop up in one direction, then give it a good push with your hands in the opposite direction, so it starts spinning around your waist on its own. Immediately begin shifting your weight forward and back, forward and back.

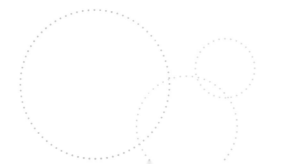

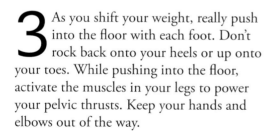

DANCE-IFY IT

Reach your arms up into the air, cross them over your chest, or place your hands on top of your head. Unclench your hands so that each finger is free, expressive, and active.

3 As you shift your weight, really push into the floor with each foot. Don't rock back onto your heels or up onto your toes. While pushing into the floor, activate the muscles in your legs to power your pelvic thrusts. Keep your hands and elbows out of the way.

4 Concentrate on sensing where your hoop touches you during its journey around your core. **Don't** *anticipate* **the hoop—***respond* **to it.** Push into it when you feel it touch you. Drive the hoop forward with your abs when you feel it rolling over your belly, and pull back firmly with your lower back when you feel the hoop rolling over your lower back.

continued ▶

▶ Pump

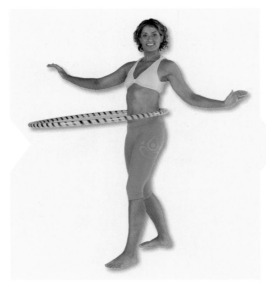

5 Use the same amount of force in pushing forward as when you pull backward—this will help keep the hoop on a flat plane, parallel to the ground. It may help to close your eyes so you can really focus on the feeling of pushing evenly both to the front and to the back.

6 If the hoop starts sloping to one side, it means your body is leaning in that direction. Compensate by gently leaning your upper body in the opposite direction, and the hoop should level out. Keep your head up, your shoulders back and down, and your neck and shoulders relaxed. Smile! Breathe! Within a matter of days or even hours, this basic building block of hooping will become second nature.

which way to go?

▶ Which direction does the hoop naturally take in circling your body? Is it coming around from your left side and moving clockwise? Or is it coming from your right side toward the left? I call the direction your hoop instinctively takes your **INFLOW**. Later you'll learn to experiment with the opposite direction, which I call the **OUTFLOW**. For now, just know that it makes no difference which way you naturally hoop. Just roll with it. The instructions for every move in the book are worded to help you into your natural **OUTFLOW** by using "the hand holding the hoop" or the "direction the hoop is rotating" as reference points, rather than "right" or "left."

contact
POINTS

When the hoop rolls around your body, it consistently makes "first contact" with two points on your body. I call these **CONTACT POINTS**. If your hoop rotates to your left, one of your **CONTACT POINTS** is behind your right hip and the other is in front of your left hip. If your hoop rotates to your right, one Point is behind your left hip while the other is in front of your right hip. Why is this important? If you focus on these spots and push into the

hoop precisely at your **CONTACT POINTS**, you will reduce the amount of energy needed to keep the hoop in orbit. This efficiency allows you to focus on dancing and moving other parts of your body.
CONTACT POINTS also run up your arms and down your legs. When you learn to hoop on your arms and legs, being able to push with precision from your **CONTACT POINTS** will be a huge help.

● = **CONTACT POINTS**
When Your Hoop Goes to the Left

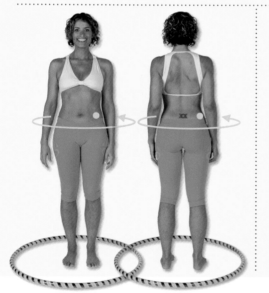

● = **CONTACT POINTS**
When Your Hoop Goes to the Right

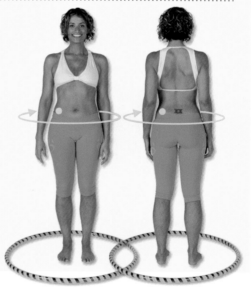

Recovery Methods

How fabulously exhilarating: The hoop is already spinning around your body! You're a superstar. It's not falling! It's not falling! And then it . . . falls. You are not alone: *Everyone* drops the hoop. So you pick it up, get it going, it's going . . . and it falls again. Don't get discouraged. Promise yourself you will succeed—and you will.

In HoopGirl classes, we say the sound of a hoop clattering to the ground is the *sound of celebration*! It means you are learning something new. When a hoop falls in class, we give a thumbs-up, wink, or hoot in encouragement. This helps everyone lighten up and enjoy learning. So keep smiling, breathe deeply, and be patient with yourself.

You can choose how you think about yourself: You're valiant, a winner, a warrior princess—seriously! The hoop—like the people around you—responds to how you hold yourself. It believes you when you say you will succeed, and will prove you right.

And there's good news! Here are three easy ways to get the hoop back up to your waist when you feel it beginning to fall.

Play with all three approaches, and then mix and match until you find the best solution for yourself. If it works, do it! For example, you may speed up, squat, and turn in quick succession. Just keep that baby spinning.

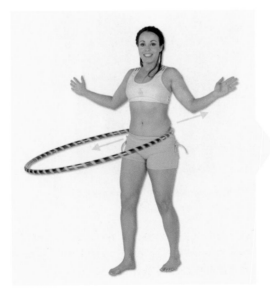

1 SPEED UP Increase the pace at which you're shifting your weight back and forth to double- or triple-time, until your hips are a blur of motion. Use power from your feet and legs to increase your pace. The hoop will naturally move up your body when you pump it at higher frequencies.

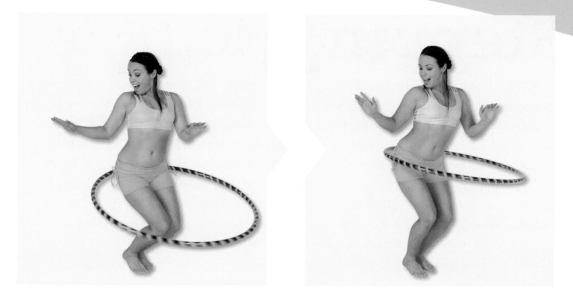

2 **SQUAT AND SHIMMY** Bend your knees and squat down to "catch" the hoop and shimmy it onto your waist. Straighten back up and immediately begin the forward and back motion of PUMP. This needs to be done in one swift motion.

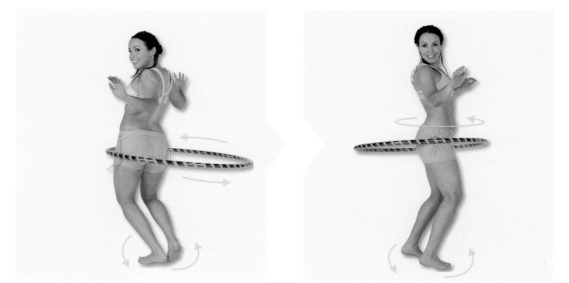

3 **TURN** Turn your body in the same direction that the hoop is moving (see pages 28–29). As you turn within the hoop, the hoop's own rotation will slow, and you can bring it back under control. Immediately resume your forward and back push-pull.

Stepping

As soon as you've stabilized the hoop's orbit around your waist, it's time to get those feet in motion. Start with baby steps—literally. With each step you take, pause afterward to regain the steady PUMP of the hoop on a flat plane around your core.

Your hoop is amazingly responsive to any change in your posture. Just shifting your weight from one foot to the other impacts the hoop's rotation. At first, anything you do with your feet will likely knock the hoop down to the ground. Just pick it up and keep going. It won't take long before you can PUMP and walk at the same time.

Keep your shoulders back and down and your head up (chin parallel to the floor) as you experiment with some basic stances and footwork.

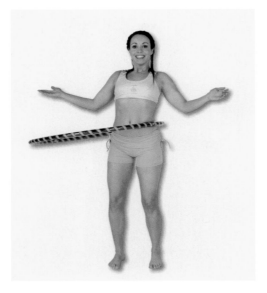

1 **STABILIZE** Stand with your feet parallel, rather than the one foot forward–one foot back, and PUMP. Your feet remain on the floor as you thrust your hips forward and back into the hoop.

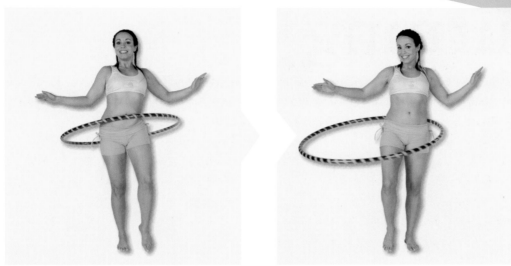

2 SHIFT YOUR WEIGHT

a. As you Pump, shift all your weight to your right foot, using your left toes just to keep balance.

b. Return to standing with your feet flat on the floor and your weight evenly distributed.

c. Shift all your weight to your left foot.

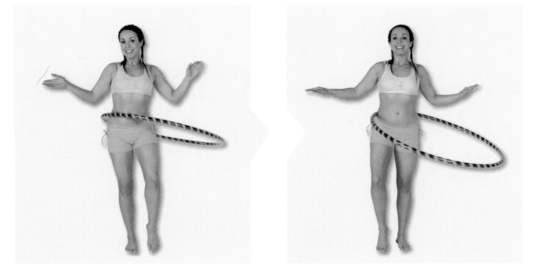

3 STEP-TOUCH

a. Continue to Pump as you step to the right with your right foot, and touch your left foot to your right.

b. Step left with your left foot, and touch with your right.

c. Step-touch-step-touch continuously side to side.

Turning

Turn your body with small, slow steps in the same direction as the hoop is moving. Practice until you can turn smoothly. It is the key to many moves you'll learn later, like the FLOAT, SNAKE, and SPUNK.

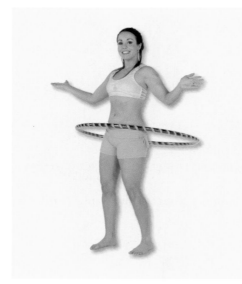

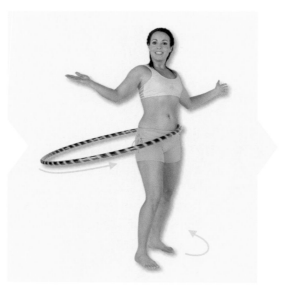

1 Start in the basic PUMP stance (one foot forward, one foot back). PUMP throughout.

2 To turn your body in the direction the hoop is turning, lead with the foot on the same side as the direction of the hoop's spin. In other words, if your hoop is rotating to the left, start turning with your left foot.

a tip for triumph

▶ Wait to step when the opening of the hoop appears in front of you; otherwise, you may knock the hoop out of orbit.

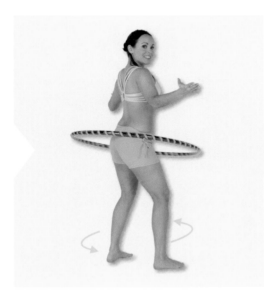

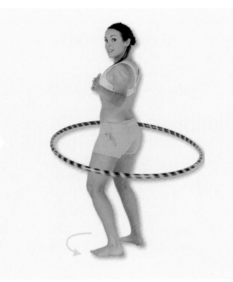

3 Stabilize the hoop in PUMP before attempting another step. When you're ready, take another tiny step to turn your body again. Imagine you are the earth rotating on its axis, with your hoop as the orbit of the moon. Both of you are spinning in the same direction.

4 Keep your head up and practice until you can walk smoothly in a circle inside your hoop as it rotates you in PUMP.

• Because turning your body contributes its own momentum, it actually enables the hoop to move around you more slowly.

Turning is *"the honey that makes everything sweeter"* in hooping! It allows your body to surrender to flow and create smooth transitions.

Easing Back Pain and Osteoporosis

DR. MICHAEL LUAN, A CHIROPRACTOR WITH A background in acupuncture and biomedical engineering, sees a lot of people with back problems. That's not surprising, given that back pain is one of the top reasons people go to the doctor. Dr. Luan regularly integrates hooping into his treatments.

Most people develop back pain from poor posture after long hours spent sitting—or worse, hunching—in front of computers and televisions. Stress and anxiety contribute to the problem. "Our day-to-day anxieties and stress cause our physiology to go into 'fear pattern'. We tuck our tails and bunch our butts, locking up the sacrum and the coccyx," says Dr. Luan. "In doing all this, we lose mobility of our hips and that is at the root of a lot of the back pain I encounter in patients."

Dr. Luan encourages hooping as a key to restoring hip mobility in his clients, helping them to unwind and unlock. "Hooping allows correct muscle sequencing, which reestablishes the balance of the load on your spine, which in turn diminishes pain and increases flexibility." In other words, the act of moving your hips fluidly shakes you out of the unhealthy ways your back muscles and bones have cemented into place from bad habits over time, so that your spine can recalibrate—back to its proper healthy position.

He also uses hooping with patients suffering from osteoporosis and its precursor, osteopenia. In these conditions, the bones lose their minerals and become brittle. "What actually causes bones to demineralize is muscular contraction," he explains. "To counteract that, you need uniform motion that works all the muscles around the spine. Hooping achieves this." He points out that the weight-bearing exercises often prescribed don't evenly work the entire circumference of muscles attached to your spine, so hooping is actually better. Your core muscles activate when you push and pull the hoop, and by being active, they keep your bones healthier. Neat!

And is there anything to watch for when starting to hoop if you already suffer from back problems? Dr. Luan recommends using common sense: "Don't hoop on bruised or inflamed areas. If your back is too bad to walk, don't hoop. But as soon as you can walk, you can get the hoop going! It's a low-impact activity that is deeply restoring."

As with all forms of exercise, to keep your lower back from being strained, allow your abdominal muscles to do a lot of work. A good way to make sure your abs are engaging is to suck them in, drawing your belly button back toward your spine. Tucking your tail by shifting your pelvis forward is another good way to protect your back.

medicine wheel

The Boundaries of Self

THE HOOP BROUGHT ME DEFINITION. It clarified the edges of my self. My whole life I've had a talent for being the person other people wanted me to be—first by learning to please my mother and teachers. At my first jobs, I had zero boundaries between work and my personal life.

In relationships, I was terribly skilled at fitting myself to the desires of my partner. Then the day would come when I'd realize I wasn't fulfilled, and I'd blame him or her for not reading me better. I don't remember thinking that people would like me less if I was myself, but I remember feeling certain that people loved me absolutely when I fashioned myself to their liking.

In striving to live up to the media's image of perfection, I was bulimic from age sixteen to twenty-six. I starved myself and binged and starved, exercised fanatically, and then binged and worked out some more, in never-ending cycles that revolved around food and consumed many of my waking hours.

In the end, I looked the part, acted the part, and got the parts: good daughter, good assistant, good wife.

At the end of my three-year marriage, I sustained an injury to my left lower back and hip area that made my bone shear upward and ripped muscle tissue so that mere walking became painful.

Then a friend took me to a hooping class at a San Francisco dance studio. Once I got the knack of keeping the hoop around my middle, it made me smile and it made me sweat. Then it became more. I found it meditative to bump the hoop in rhythm with the music. I felt safe encircled by my hoop.

The hoop impacts your body twice each rotation. Since I'm predisposed to hooping to my right, it touches me on the front of my right hip and the back of my left hip—there where I was injured. My chiropractor says it's the best thing I could do for myself, providing continuous massage of the mass of scar tissue. But more important, the sensation is a reminder of my physical boundaries—*these are the edges of Ariane,* the hoop whispers as it circles me. It makes me feel whole, independent, strong, and self-confident.

Spending so much time isolated within my hoop has enabled me to finally hear my desires and needs. I no longer have to rely on seeing myself reflected in the eyes of other people to believe in myself.

Hooping renders me radiant; and though I hear that confirmed from other people, I don't need them to tell me. I feel it.

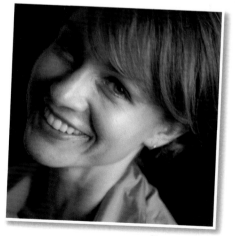

Name: Ariane
Occupation: Writer

THE MOVES

Explore Your Core

TONING YOUR TUMMY & ENERGIZING YOUR CENTER

Core strength, core stability, core rhythms . . . it seems like you can't open the pages of a magazine or turn on a television without encountering this hot region of the body. Why all the hype? Well, take a look at yourself: Your head, arms, and legs all stem from your torso. To move through life, your center needs to be strong!

You've probably heard that yoga and Pilates are excellent activities for working the core. Now you can add hooping to the list. It works the entire entourage of core muscles, large and small. PUMP is the quintessential core hooping move—and you've already mastered it! In this chapter you'll learn to move the hoop higher and lower on your torso, and then bring it onto diagonal angles. Each of these skills focuses on different parts of your core.

The biggest difference between hooping and other top-recommended core builders? You'll giggle while you hoop. (And laughter is another way to exercise your abdominals!)

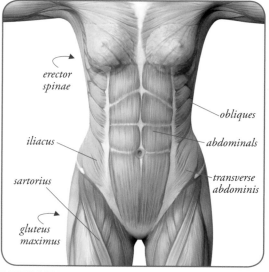

erector
spinae

obliques

iliacus

abdominals

sartorius

transverse
abdominis

gluteus
maximus

Core Muscles

Just as your abdominals go well beyond the "six-pack muscle," your core involves a lot more than your abdominals. There's the trio of muscles that extends along your neck to your lower back (*erector spinae*). Under them there are the *multifidus,* which allow your spine to move around. Abs not quite as prominent as the six-pack include the *obliques* and the deep-seated TVA (*transverse abdominis*) muscle. You feel the TVA contract when you cough. Then there's the whole crew around your hips and butt, like a squadron of gladiators (*iliacus, sartorius, gluteus*

maximus, to name a few). They allow you to sit, bend, and walk.

Together, these muscles stabilize your spine, pelvis, hips, abdomen—even your legs and shoulders. They provide the foundation for standing upright, for shifting your weight, and for pretty much any movement you can think of, even a modest action like answering your cell phone. "When core muscles are strong and toned, they work together to support your spine and to stabilize and preserve your posture, which reduces your risk for back injuries," says fitness expert Jorge Cruise, author of *The 12-Second Sequence.* For optimal agility and total body strength, both your deep and superficial core muscles need to be fortified.

Inner Essence

Some cultures believe your absolute core is located even deeper than in your muscles and bones. In Chinese medicine, the fundamental life force energy is called *chi* (pronounced "chee"), also known in other cultures as *prana.* Chinese philosopher Zhuang Zi of the fourth century B.C. wrote: "Human beings are born [because

Mobilizing the chi

of] the accumulation of chi. When it accumulates there is life. When it dissipates there is death. . . . This vital force is the key animating element in any living thing."

Chi is the basis of Chinese medicine, acupuncture, Shiatsu, chiropractic, and Ayurvedic medicine, as well as movement forms such as yoga and tai chi. It underlies martial arts such as aikido, which translates to "the way of unifying with life energy." Chi is even the basis of feng shui, a type of interior design based on balancing energy. The foundation of all these practices is belief in the existence of an animating energy that can be directed and increased in order to optimize health and well-being.

In the body, the home of chi is in the abdomen, three finger widths below the navel and two finger widths behind it. Core hooping provides a constant, gentle yet firm massage of this area. The main pathways for the movement of chi are called *meridians*,

Hooping and Acupressure

ARTURO PEAL, AN EXPERT IN CHINESE MEDICINE, anatomy, and kinesiology, recommends hooping to his clients primarily for unblocking chi. It's a common diagnosis in our culture, he says, "where people don't move enough physically or emotionally." Symptoms include restricted movement along the sides of the torso, severe PMS, depression, and a weakened immune system. The best cure for stagnation of chi is simply to get yourself, your blood, and your lymph moving, he says. "Movement in the hips as with salsa or hooping is ideal."

Peal points out that "like acupressure treatments, the hoop stimulates many vital points, impacting the most important organs of the body." Around the hips, on the back side of the body, the hoop's pressure impacts the bladder, the kidneys, the large intestine, and the points that relate to low back pain. On the front of the body, it reaches the stomach, kidneys, liver, and spleen—and the locations of many points used for digestive and reproductive issues.

medicine wheel

When the hoop rolls over the back of your hand, it can impact some of the points that have powerful systemic effects, particularly to treat pain (such as headaches and toothaches), insomnia, and anxiety, as well as local pain in that region from carpal tunnel and repetitive stress injuries.

There are even special acupressure hoops for sale in Asian markets. These are covered with bumps that are intended to increase the pressure on vital points. Unfortunately, there have been many reports of injuries caused by sustained hooping using these specialized hoops. Neither Dr. Peal nor I can recommend them. As he says, a regular smooth hoop works just fine. Don't mess with simple perfection!

Your Core Score

ASSESS THE STRENGTH AND STABILITY OF YOUR core by taking this simple test, developed by long-time track and field coach Brian Mackenzie. Someone with a powerful core will be able to remain balanced while supporting her entire weight on one arm and the opposite leg while the other arm and leg are held in the air.

1 Get into the Plank position: Starting facedown on the floor, lift your body off the ground onto your elbows and toes. Your elbows should be under your shoulders with your forearms resting on the floor, your hands relaxed. Your toes should be curled under so they face forward. Your abs should be engaged, your neck and shoulders relaxed, and your back flat.

2 Lift your right arm off the floor, extending it forward and holding it in the air for fifteen seconds.

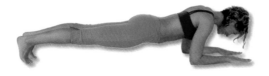

3 Return your right arm to the floor, and lift your left arm off the ground. Hold for fifteen seconds.

4 Return your left arm and lift your right leg off the floor. Hold for fifteen seconds.

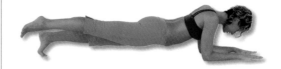

5 Return your right leg and lift your left leg. Hold for fifteen seconds.

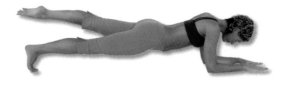

6 Now lift your left leg and your right arm at the same time. Hold them aloft for fifteen seconds.

7 Return them to the floor, then lift your right leg and left arm together. Hold for fifteen seconds.

8 Return to the starting Plank position and hold it for thirty more seconds.

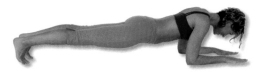

How Far Did You Get?

▶ **To 3:**
Aluminum Core.
Hey, I'm shiny.
What more do you want?

▶ **To 5:**
Platinum Core.
I'm strong enough for precious gems . . .

▶ **To 8:**
Titanium Core.
I'm invincible. Watch out world!

You can repeat this exercise as often as you like. It's a great way to chart your progress as you increase the power of your core muscles. In addition to measuring it, this test is also a great exercise to *build* your core strength.

each of which correspond to the twelve major organs and most of which are located in the abdomen and pelvic region. When the hoop rolls over your core, it also stimulates these pathways, just as acupuncture and acupressure do.

the bootylicious
PLAYLIST

Hip-hop specially engineered for powerful and sassy core maneuvers . . .

1. **HIPS DON'T LIE**   Shakira (ft. Wyclef Jean)
2. **LOSE MY BREATH**   Destiny's Child
3. **MY HUMPS**   Black Eyed Peas
4. **MILKSHAKE**   Kelis
5. **TAKE CONTROL**   Amerie
6. **WIND IT UP**   Gwen Stefani
7. **JUMP ON**   Thara (ft. Fat Man Scoop)
8. **CUPID SHUFFLE**   Cupid
9. **FERGALICIOUS**   Fergie
10. **THE ANTHEM**   Pitbull (ft. Lil Jon)

Play All the Angles

In this book I'll talk about the hoop being on three different planes: horizontal, vertical, and diagonal.

When I describe the hoop as HORIZONTAL, it should stay parallel to the ground. The classic example is PUMP. There are lots of other moves that keep the hoop in this plane, for example, WILDWEST, HORIZONTAL WHISPER, and CAROUSEL. Note that horizontal moves can take place at any level or height—you can pass the hoop around your ankles in a low-to-the-ground variation of NECTAR, or at the opposite extreme you can keep the hoop circling as high above your head as you can reach in WILDWEST.

A VERTICAL move keeps the hoop perpendicular to

amplify
YOUR WILL

The jaw is connected to the hips by a meridian. Because of this, the looser your hips become, the more easily your jaw moves. (In other words, loose hips loosen lips.) In the metaphorical sense, a more mobile jaw expresses thoughts more clearly when you speak.

Practice yelling "YES!" and then "NO!" for several minutes while hooping in PUMP. Many people find it hard to say "NO," but doing so can build your assertiveness and determination. And saying "YES" to your beauty or your worthiness when you are feeling less than spectacular is a healthy challenge.

the ground. Verticality is generally achieved when the hoop is held in one or both hands, off the body. (*Note:* Some acrobatic hoopers can keep the hoop in the vertical plane using their legs or feet as well.) A classic vertical move is SWISH, but there are a ton of others, such as TOSS, GARTER, and SPARKLE.

There are also DIAGONAL moves, in which the hoop is somewhere between the horizontal and vertical planes. These include the moves you're about to learn: BOOTY BUMP, LIMBO, and BARREL ROLL. (*Note:* Some moves in which the hoop is "carried"

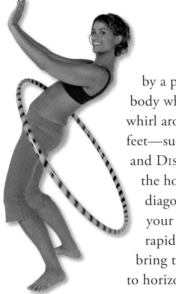

by a part of your body while you whirl around on your feet—such as LIBRA and DISCO—put the hoop on the diagonal until your footwork is rapid enough to bring the hoop up to horizontal.)

Getting Slanty

Bringing the hoop onto a diagonal angle feels satisfying, looks cool, and provides an amazing workout for your abdomen and lower back. That's because the hoop provides weighted resistance against your core muscles as you lean forward or back to push the hoop onto a diagonal angle. Maintaining the angle requires precision and strength! Because you also need to lift your heels off the

"Hooping has been an amazing cardio workout. Now, four months later, my abs look like they did ten years ago!"

—Marci, 56

ground in these moves when you push into the hoop, they stimulate your calf and thigh muscles as well.

To keep your lower back from being strained during diagonal moves, be sure to make your abdominal muscles do the brunt of the work. Remember to contract your abs and pull your belly button toward your spine to make sure your abs are engaged.

As for specific angles to shoot for—see how far toward vertical your hoop can get. A beginning hooper usually accomplishes a hoop angle closer to forty-five degrees, while, with practice, the hoop will get closer and closer to vertical, or about eighty degrees.

LIMBO and BOOTY BUMP are some saucy moves . . . they involve blatant pelvic thrusting! Release your inhibitions as you go diagonal.

The diagonal becomes vertical

Churning

Accelerate the hoop's pace in PUMP to supersonic speeds for a set period of time, punctuated by breaks at slow speeds to recover.

NOTE: Have a timer or a clock with a second hand visible nearby.

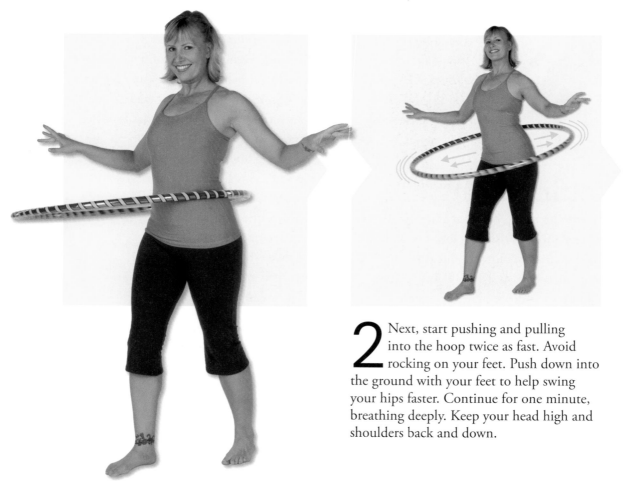

2 Next, start pushing and pulling into the hoop twice as fast. Avoid rocking on your feet. Push down into the ground with your feet to help swing your hips faster. Continue for one minute, breathing deeply. Keep your head high and shoulders back and down.

1 Start in PUMP. Spend two minutes getting into the natural rhythm of your hoop.

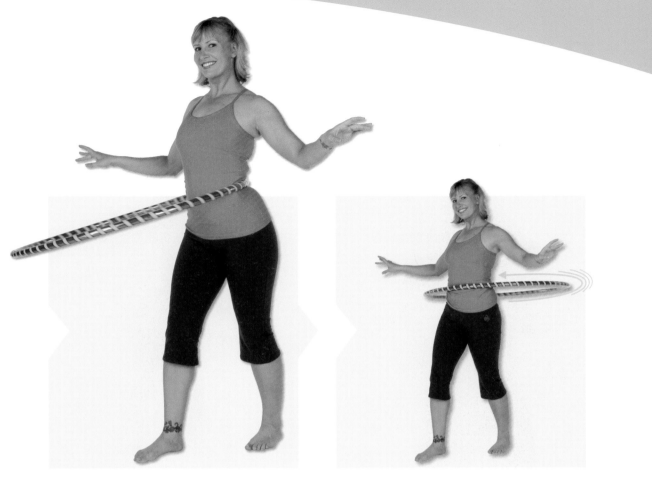

3 After one minute has passed, slow to a regular PUMP to give yourself a break for about thirty seconds.

4 Return to CHURNING with warp-speed rotations. Continue alternating speeds until you feel warm and tingly, about four to six reps. CHURNING is an excellent exercise you can do in reps for strength training or to warm your muscles before other core moves.

Booty Blitz

Go low! Rotating on the horizontal plane, the hoop rolls over the buttocks and the front of the pelvis below the hips.

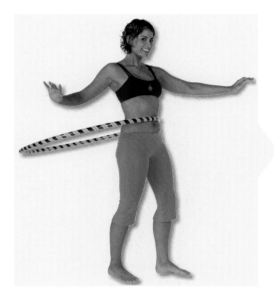

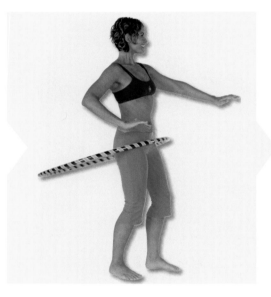

1 Get the hoop going in Pump. Begin reducing the hoop's speed by slowing the forward-back swing of your hips. The hoop will start to sink toward the floor.

2 As soon as you feel the hoop roll onto your buns, get fast and assertive with your forward-back, push-pull movement. The hoop should be below your hip bones. Push into the hoop right above your pubic bone. Your hips are a blur of motion, like the wings of a hummingbird.

a tip for triumph

▶ If your movements are too fast, the hoop may pop back up to your waist. If this happens, keep breathing and simply slow your hips so the hoop moves down again and pick up the speed. If you are hooping too slowly, the hoop will fall. If this happens, use a Recovery Method (page 24).

DANCE-IFY IT

March in place, which pumps your gluteal (butt) muscles and creates a more defined surface for the hoop's percussion. Meanwhile, dance with your upper body by extending your arms out to each side and turning your head left and right.

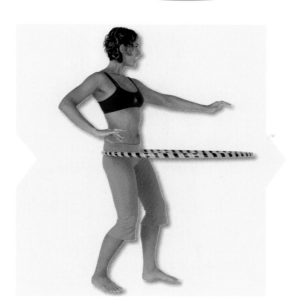

3 As the hoop rolls over your butt, pull back, leading with your tailbone. You should feel a nice massage on your sciatic nerves. Keep your shoulders back and down and your head high, looking straight ahead. Breathe.

4 Push firmly into the floor with both the balls and heels of your feet. Avoid rocking up onto your toes or back onto your heels. Keeping your feet connected allows you to push against the resistance of the ground, and thereby increase the pace and precision of your hip motions.

Pulse

Shimmy the hoop up and down the torso continuously with side-to-side movements while keeping the hoop on a horizontal plane. This move is an awesome way to warm you up on a cold morning in the park!

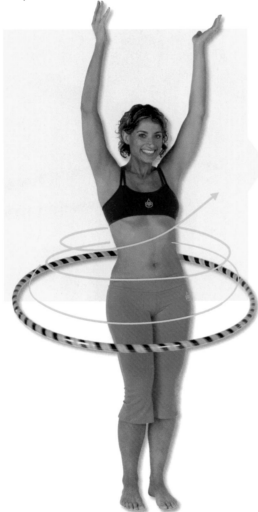

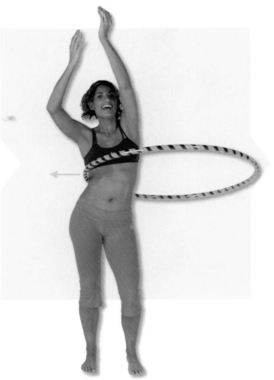

2 Shift your awareness to the points where the hoop is touching you on the sides of your body. Now start moving your torso side to side by pushing left and right with your chest, until your movements are 100 percent side to side. Deepen your breath to maintain the brisk movements.

1 Get the hoop going in PUMP. Lift your arms out of the way by reaching up toward the ceiling so your elbows are at shoulder height or above. Quicken the pace of your push-pull movements.

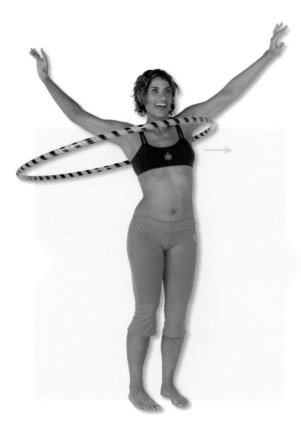

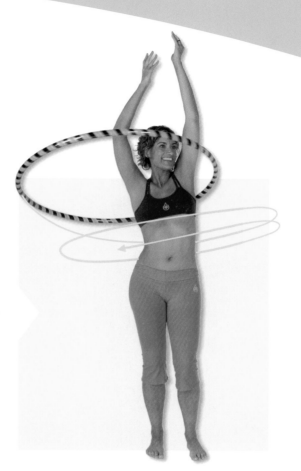

3 Continue with exaggerated movements of your upper torso to keep the hoop rising up your body. The best way to describe the movement is wiggling all over like a wet noodle. Instead of your hips, a new set of muscles should engage in your upper abdomen. The hoop may wobble or shift back down, but continue with your quick side-to-side pushing to shimmy the hoop up your ribs.

4 Continue until the hoop reaches just underneath your armpits. Keep the hoop up there as long as you can, then let it move back down your torso into PUMP. When you're ready, energize your core and shimmy the hoop up again. Mastery means you can fluidly raise and lower the hoop repeatedly.

• Return to PULSE again and again as a regular practice to build amazing core stamina. The more chill the rest of your body can remain, breathing deeply and relaxing your facial muscles, the better.

Limbo

Remember dancing lower and lower under the pole in a game of Limbo? Your body had to be practically parallel to the floor to stay in the game. This move uses that same core strength to lean back and push the hoop up with the front of your abs, so the hoop slopes diagonally upward in front of you.

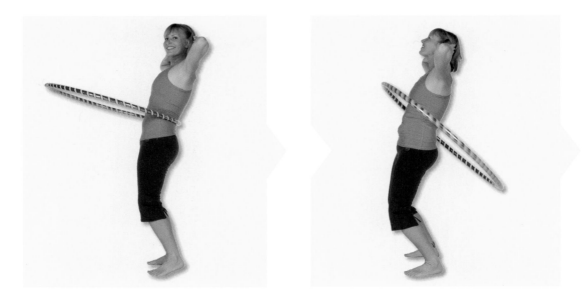

1 Start in PUMP. Engage your abdominals and lean back slightly, tilting the front of your pelvis upward. Instead of pushing forward and back, when you feel the hoop roll over your abs, concentrate all your efforts on *pushing up* toward the sky. To keep your arms out of the hoop's way, cross them on your chest or put them behind your head.

2 Look up! When you tilt your head to look directly skyward, you reorient your entire torso so that it faces up. The goal is to bring your upper body into as parallel a position with the floor as possible while still engaging your abs. Keep breathing so your face and jaw stay relaxed.

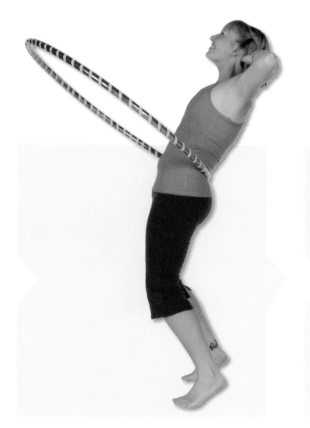

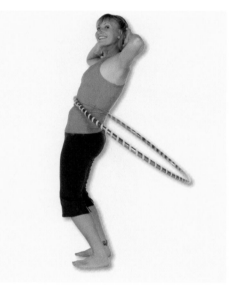

3 Create an up-and-down bounce by rising onto the balls of your feet and down on your heels over and over again, like you've got springs in your heels. The bounce may cause you to travel forward slightly. This is fine. The balls of your feet are always connected to the ground while your *heels* go up and down.

4 As your legs thrust you upward, continue to push the hoop up with your belly each time it rolls over your front. Your back is not doing any work to push the hoop. Continue until your thigh and core muscles ask for a break, and return to PUMP.

a tip for triumph

▶ If your hoop slopes off to one side, alter your posture by stepping forward with the leg opposite the slope. This should return the hoop to a straight path across your belly.

Booty Bump

This move is the reverse of LIMBO: Lean forward and push the hoop up with your lower back, so it slopes diagonally down in front of you.

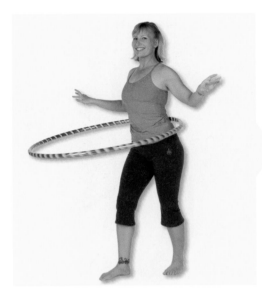
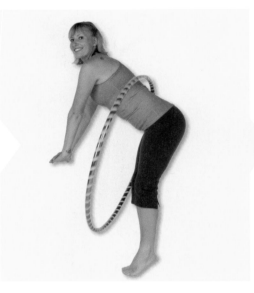

1 Start in PUMP. Lean your upper body slightly forward toward the floor, arching your back slightly and tilting your pelvis forward. Keep your arms up and out of the way.

2 When you feel the hoop roll over the small of your back, rise onto the balls of your feet and lift your heels to help pop the hoop up. Let your heels bounce down again and again. The bouncing may cause you to travel backward slightly. That's OK.

verbalize

▶ While in PUMP, say "now" each time the hoop makes contact with your lower back. Keep saying it out loud, maintaining the rhythm, as you tilt your pelvis forward to launch the hoop onto its angle. This can help you master the timing of when to lift up your heels and thrust upward with your lower back.

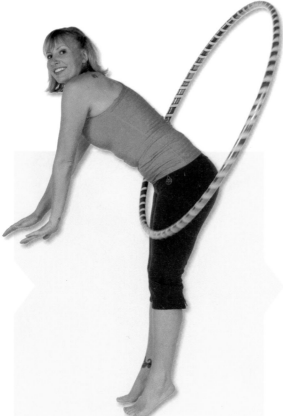

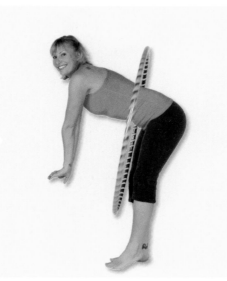

3 Sync up the thrust from your feet and the small of your back with the rhythm of the hoop. Look straight ahead instead of at the floor, and remember to breathe. Pretend you're a marionette with strings attached to the back of your hip bones, which are being pulled straight up.

4 If your hoop slopes off to one side, gently alter your posture by stepping forward with the leg opposite the slope. If your hoop is sloping so much that it hits your knees, stand a bit more upright. If you feel the hoop slipping down your buttocks, take a small hop backward to bring it up higher on your back.

Barrel Roll

This move combines LIMBO and BOOTY BUMP into one seamless rotation by turning the body over and over on itself while keeping the hoop on its diagonal angle.

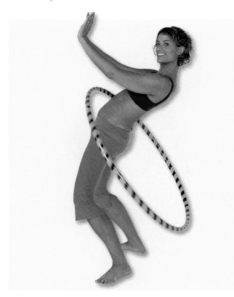

1 Get the hoop into LIMBO, with a strong diagonal angle. Keep your arms up and out of your hoop's way.

2 Lift the foot on the *opposite* side of the body from the direction the hoop is traveling. As you lift your foot, pivot on the other foot to flip your body over so you are facing downward.

a tip for triumph

▶ You need to be able to stand on one foot and pivot on it—that is, to rotate your body by swiveling on that foot without taking it off the ground. It helps to practice first without the hoop. "Flip" your body over (a 180-degree turn) by pivoting on one foot.

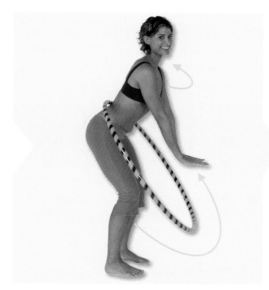

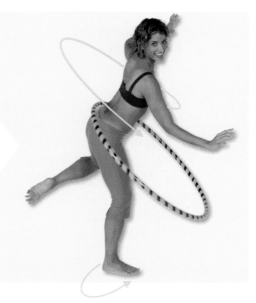

3 Keep your face up even though your torso is leaning forward! Then standing on both feet with your weight equally distributed, do BOOTY BUMP. When you are ready to roll again, lift the foot on the *same* side of the body as the direction the hoop is traveling. (If the hoop is rotating to the left, lift the left foot.)

4 As you lift up that foot, pivot on the other foot and turn your body again so you end up facing upward. Then stand on both feet with your weight equally distributed and LIMBO.

• Maintain distinct angles, by vigorously popping the hoop up into LIMBO and down into BOOTY BUMP before and after your BARREL ROLL.

• Keep your torso nearly parallel to the floor while in LIMBO and BOOTY BUMP. With practice, your BARREL ROLL will become smoother and the rotation of your body more rapid.

Getting My Groove Back

TWO YEARS AFTER MOVING TO A NEW CITY, I still didn't know my away around. I hadn't ventured out much and was stuck in a rut—working long hours and getting home in time to just make dinner and go to bed, only to start all over again the next morning. I felt like a robot. Where was my mojo? I had always been the life of the party. Now I couldn't even remember what fun felt like.

So I decided to do something that would get my sluggish body moving. I thought about belly dancing or pole dancing to revive my dry bones and make me feel alive again. Then I came across hooping classes.

When I first started hooping I felt like I had zero rhythm or coordination. I must have dropped the hoop a zillion times. I can't imagine what the people who live below me thought I was doing. But I gradually built my skills and my confidence. Now I love getting out and meeting up with other local hoopers, with their very different personalities, various hooping styles, and new tricks to share. It's an amazing social outlet.

So, there, Austin Powers, I found my mojo! My new alter ego is Catwoman! I mean, it's one thing to be told that you're sexy, but it's an altogether different thing to really *feel* sexy. With hooping, I feel it. And, incidentally, my husband feels it too. He's always eager to see my moves and my exuberance. He's thrilled to have the "old Monica" back. So am I.

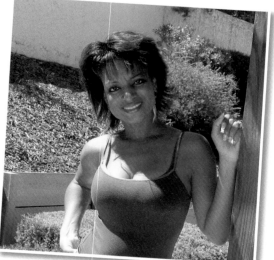

Name: Monica
Occupation: Finance

Core Beliefs

Core strength can be more profound than muscles and even chi—it can also refer to our deepest-held beliefs about ourselves and the world. Everyone has core beliefs— these are the answers to the big questions such as "Who am I?," "What is life for?," and "What is my purpose?" They are the lenses through which we view life.

Your beliefs influence your hooping! They can cause you either to keep faith or get frustrated every time you drop your hoop. They affect whether you decide to show your skin or cover it up. They influence whether you share hooping with everyone you know or keep it to yourself. They create your drive to learn more—or the decision to throw in the towel.

Somatic movement therapists believe that the body, mind, and spirit are one continuous whole, which means that your core beliefs can be influenced by movement, and vice versa. So not only do your beliefs impact your hooping, your hooping can actually impact your beliefs! Be open to the possibility that freeing up your hips may free your mind too.

Become aware of what story you're living: You have the power to change it. Take a moment to assess which of the following statements resonate with you. You might want to write in your journal about beliefs you'd like to change.

WHAT'S YOUR TRUTH?

I can do anything.	This is hard. Life is hard!
I deserve love and happiness.	I'm not good enough.
I am a good person.	There is something wrong with me.
I can learn to master any new skill.	I'm bad at _____. I just can't do it.
My life is a series of miracles!	Bad things just happen to me.
I'm young at heart and full of energy.	I'm getting old and out of shape.
I'm surrounded by community.	I'm alone and I don't fit in.
There is enough for us all to enjoy.	There's not enough to go around.
I am safe and secure and all is well.	It's not safe!
My body is the perfect shape and size.	I'm too fat/thin.
I love the sensual beauty of my body!	Being sexy is dirty and bad.

THE MOVES

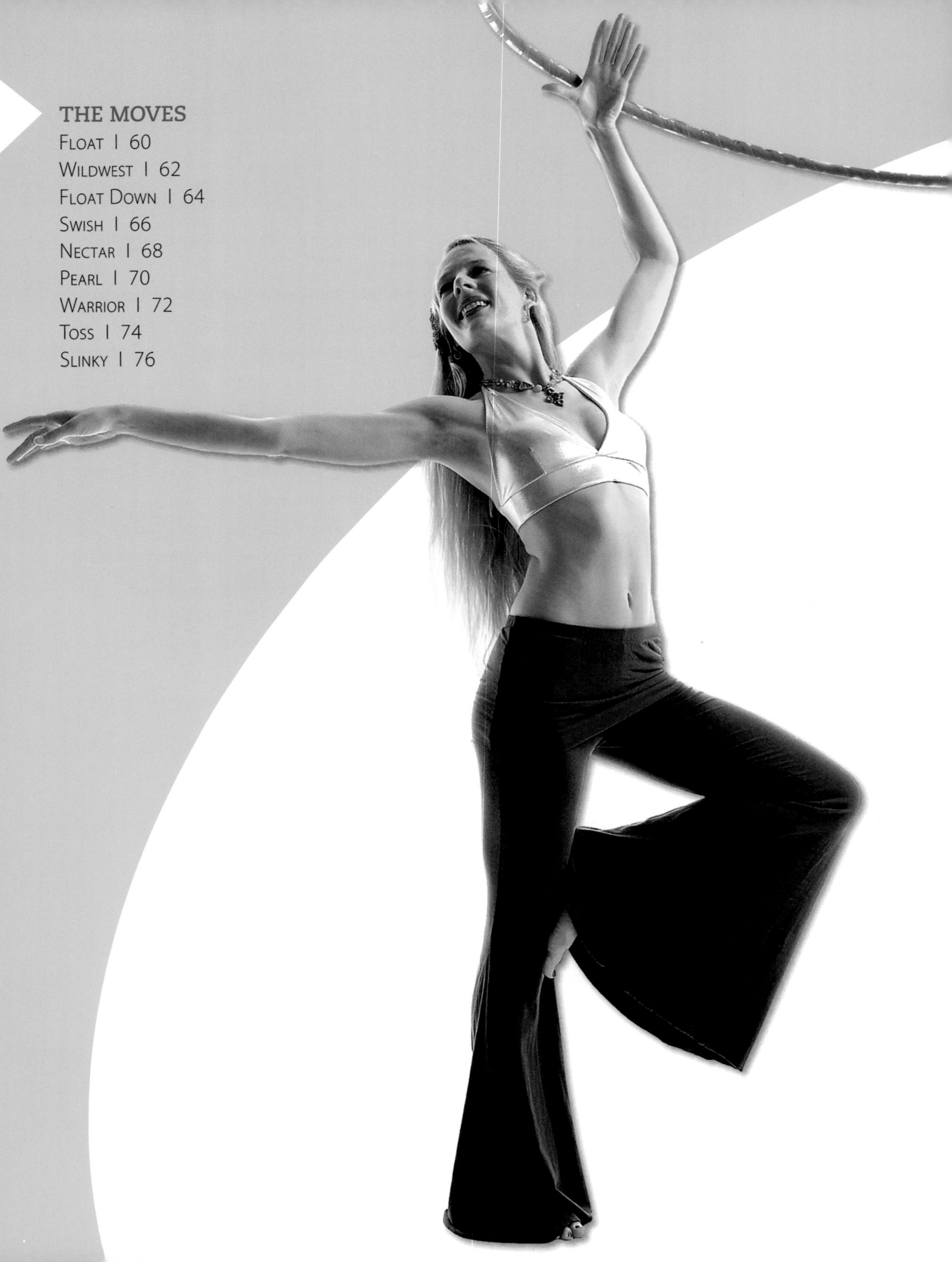

A Call to Arms

GETTING BUFF BICEPS, TONED TRICEPS & WRISTS OF STEEL

When you mention hooping, most people think of the hoop circling around the waist. It comes as a shock when they learn how fantastic hooping can be for the shoulders, arms, wrists, and hands too! But it's true.

There are a ton of moves where the hoop is not on your core—instead you use your hands and arms to move it around. These are called *off-body* moves. There are also a few *transitional* moves in which you use your hands to take the hoop from your core to an off-body position (as in FLOAT) or to bring it back onto your body (as in FLOAT DOWN). With these moves, it takes only a few minutes before you feel the resistance provided by the weight of the hoop in your deltoids, biceps, triceps, forearms, and wrists.

Off-body moves specifically exercise the arms and shoulders, but remember that even while hooping on the core, you can and should *mobilize* your arms.

You can swing, flutter, and punch your arms expressively and rhythmically while core hooping. If you've had any experience with a form of dance or martial arts, take those arm movements and pair them with PUMP or BOOTY BLITZ, for example. As any dancer can tell you, sustained arm and hand movements give you an incredible workout without ever needing to get near a pair of dumbbells.

Whether you are heaven-bent on firming up your upper arms, or even if you take your upper-body fitness for granted, physical therapists say it's important to regularly challenge the area. People who don't can lose the ability to lift, push, and pull objects in their later years. Strong arms will help you live an active and independent life for the long haul. So reach out, grab your hoop, and sound the call to arms!

"It's incredible how toned and sculpted my arms have become from hooping. They add such a beautiful and graceful element to my dance as they naturally float out and away from my body."

—Anne, 32

Shoulders and Elbows and Wrists, Oh My!

These three joints in and around the arms play significant roles while you're hooping off-body.

WRISTS. These gateways between your hands and arms are powerful. Your wrists can help balance your body, such as when you hold on to a handrail, and can even bear your full weight, for instance, when you do a handstand. Many off-body moves require and develop a LOT of wrist strength. Make sure you practice these in small doses so you don't strain your wrists. If your wrists seem weak, you might consider consulting a medical practitioner about wearing a wrist brace or taking a calcium, flaxseed oil, and/or glucosamine/chondroitin/MSM supplement. You can also experiment with a feather-weight hoop.

ELBOWS. These guys are for more than pushing people out of the way! Hooping deepens your appreciation for the elegant hinges that connect your upper arms and forearms. In moves like JINGLE and FLING, you'll discover that elbows are capable of expressive dance and rhythmic percussion. You'll gain awareness of the angle and height of your elbows as well as the different degrees of openness this hinge can achieve.

SHOULDERS. Shoulders take on a lot: They can carry a "chip," "the weight of the world," or a friend looking for something "to cry on." So they had better be strong! Most new hoopers need to pay attention to avoid a forward "slump" by keeping the shoulders relaxed, back, and down. When relaxed, shoulders can be more mobile. Later in the book, with the intermediate move called LIBRA (page 150), you'll learn to keep the hoop riding on the surface of your shoulder.

Absolutely Gripping

Before you start the off-body moves that will give your core a well-deserved rest, here's a short tutorial on positioning your hands on the hoop. In class, I encourage students to use their intuition about how and where to hold the hoop. Sometimes breaking things down like I'm about to do can make you overthink it. It blocks the way you'd naturally hold something. So skim this section, and return to it later when a certain grip stumps you.

An *Inside* grip versus an *Outside* grip.
Because the hoop is made of a round tube, the exact edges of *Outside* versus *Inside* are hard to mark. Consider most of the hoop's

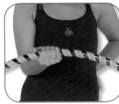 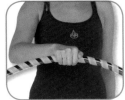

Inside grip   Outside grip

surface to be *Outside*, and just the remaining strip that is the inner surface to be *Inside*. The way you move between the inside and outside of the hoop is by loosening your grip, articulating your fingers around the hoop one at a time, and reasserting your grip on the outside of the hoop, facing in.

Keeping a solid grip on the hoop.
To practice this, hold the hoop vertically in front of you, gripping the outside of the hoop as though you were shaking hands with it. You can raise and lower the hoop without altering your grip at all.

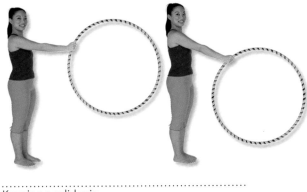

Keeping a solid grip

Twisting your wrist to change the angle or position of the hoop. To see how this feels, grip the hoop as shown, below, using your right hand. Twist your wrist ninety degrees counterclockwise. The hoop should move from the vertical plane onto the horizontal.

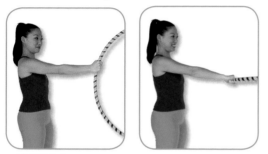

Twisting to the horizontal plane

Flipping your wrist involves one quick twist that puts your hand in the opposite position. To practice this, grip the hoop vertically in front of you as shown, below. Notice that your thumb is facing up. In one quick motion, twist 180 degrees counterclockwise. The hoop ends in the vertical plane, and your thumb is now facing down.

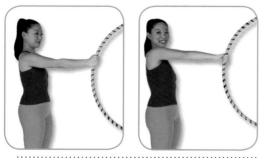

Flipping 180 degrees

Allowing the hoop to swivel in your grip. Hold the hoop on a horizontal plane, gripping from the outside, with your knuckles up and palm down. It's fine if you need to use both hands to hold the hoop—just place them close together, thumb to thumb. Now loosen your grip ever so slightly so the hoop swivels and falls to the vertical plane.

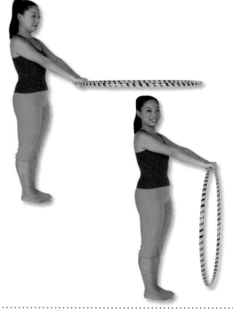

Allowing the hoop to swivel

Note: Usually, swiveling is accomplished not by *loosening* your grip, as in this example, but by exerting significant wrist strength to shift the hoop into a new position. To see how much strength this takes, try to bring the hoop back from the vertical to the horizontal by swiveling the hoop upward.

Allowing the hoop to roll over your hand and renew your grip. Often, you'll have to release your grip altogether for a moment and let the hoop roll over part of your hand (often the back of your hand, under your knuckles) before gripping it again.

Rather than thinking about these concepts in the abstract, try experimenting with them. Don't overthink it. With practice you'll learn how to grip, shift, release, and reassert your grip.

an armful of tunes
PLAYLIST

Infused with Spanish and Asian influences that invite flowing and percussive movements.

1.	**SANTA MARIA (DEL BUEN AYRE)**	Gotan Project
2.	**MAMBO NO. 5**	Perez Prado y Su Orquesta
3.	**CANTO A LA HABANA**	Bebo Valdes
4.	**SUAVEMENTE**	Elvis Crespo
5.	**LA BOQUILLA**	Ska Cubano
6.	**EL CEPILLO**	Fulanito
7.	**NAMOH NAMOH**	Daler Mehndi
8.	**RHYTHMS OF BOLLYWOOD**	Taufiq Qureshi
9.	**LA INDIA CON LA VOE (MAW TRIBIN)**	MAW (ft. India)
10.	**CHANTOS**	David Ospina

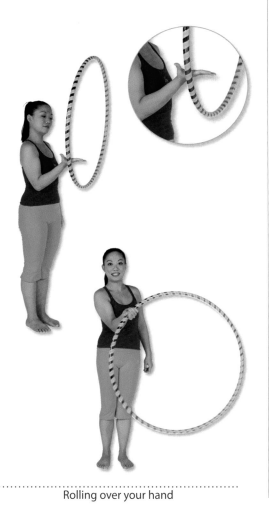

Rolling over your hand

Float

Lift the hoop from your waist to above your head on a horizontal plane. It's a graceful way to move the hoop off your core and into your hand.

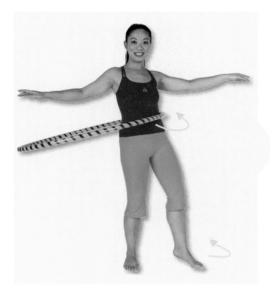

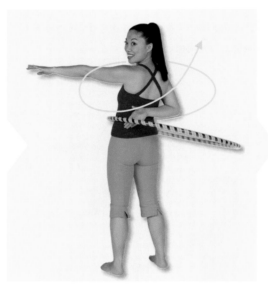

1 Start in PUMP. Slow your forward-back rocking so the hoop moves around you as slowly as possible while still orbiting your waist. Turn continuously by taking small steps in the direction of the hoop's rotation.

2 Use the hand opposite the direction the hoop is traveling (if the hoop is rotating to your left, use your right hand). Reach that hand around your back as far as possible, so it rests flush against your opposite hip. Your palm should face away from your body, with your fingers pointing down.

a tip for triumph

▶ Key to achieving this move is the unique grip switch. As you raise the hoop overhead, allow your grip to switch from the inside of the hoop, to the outside, and then back to the inside. Next, go into WILDWEST (page 62).

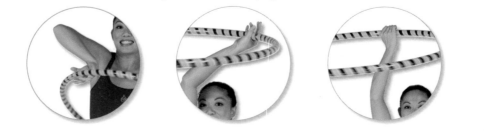

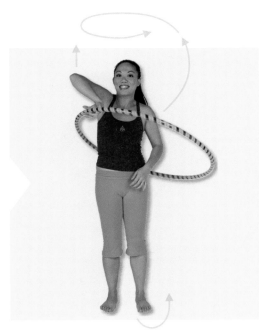

3 While still turning your body, lightly grip the hoop as it rolls over your open palm and lift the hoop up, leading with your elbow. (Turning creates time for you to lift the hoop, and allows your arm to move into a more natural position.) Allow the hoop to continue its spiraling rotation as it lifts up and around your body, like a corkscrew lifting a cork.

NOTE: Steps 3 and 4 happen quickly, in one fell swoop.

4 Bring the hoop over your head with your arm extended above you. (Keep your palm up and lead with your pinky.)

5 Once it's above your head, allow the hoop to roll over the back of your hand, switching your grip from the inside to the outside and then back to the inside.

• It's OK if your arm gets tangled with the hoop while lifting the first few times. Stay positive and keep at it.

Wildwest

Imagine you are Wonder Woman with her golden lasso and twirl the hoop horizontally above your head with one hand.

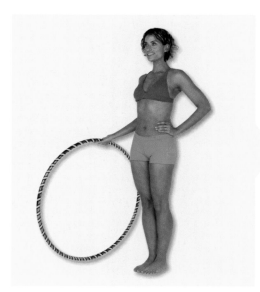

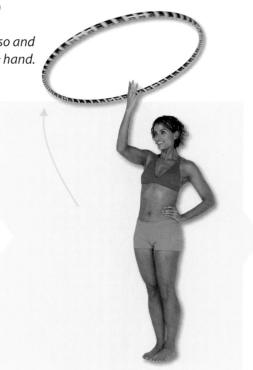

1 You can go right into WILDWEST from FLOAT or start with the hoop at your side. Lift the hoop up and overhead. Grip the hoop on the inside, with your palm facing out.

2 Engage your entire arm to swing the hoop into motion overhead.

be aware!

▶ It's important to briefly grip the hoop once each revolution! This is how you keep the hoop under control and on the horizontal. If you don't, the hoop could fly off your hand and hit the people or objects around you.

DANCE-IFY IT

Wildwest is a great move to combine with some fancy-free footwork. Experiment with martial arts kicks, squats, or lunges while in Wildwest to work your lower body too.

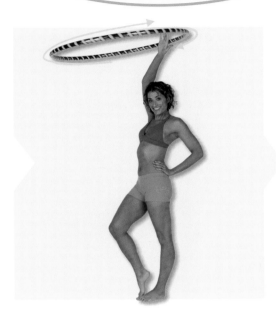

3 On each rotation of the hoop, allow the hoop to *roll over the back of your hand* (below your knuckles), briefly grip the hoop, then release the grip and push so the hoop continues its lasso twirl.

• Practice Wildwest in small doses, as the back of the hand needs to adjust to the pressure of the hoop. (A lightweight hoop is easier on your hands.) Alternate hands. It might feel awkward in your nondominant hand, but it will build dexterity and strength.

Float Down

Bring the hoop from WILDWEST back onto your core.

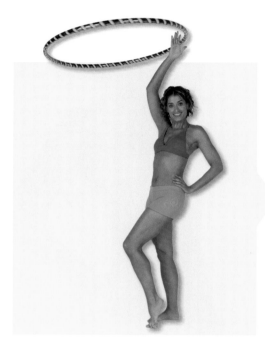

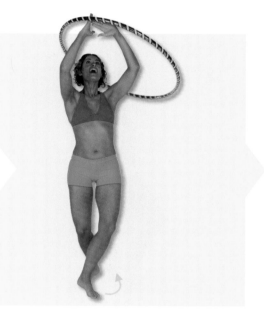

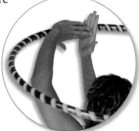

1 Start in WILDWEST. Use the same hand you used in FLOAT UP, and make sure the hoop is moving in your INFLOW (page 22). Take small continuous steps in the direction the hoop is moving to turn your body. When you're ready, let the WILDWEST hand begin to carry the hoop down over your head.

2 Place your free hand palm-out on the inside of the hoop. Your fingers should point to the side with your pinky on top as though you are shielding your eyes from the sun. Both hands should now be in contact with the hoop, just an inch or two apart.

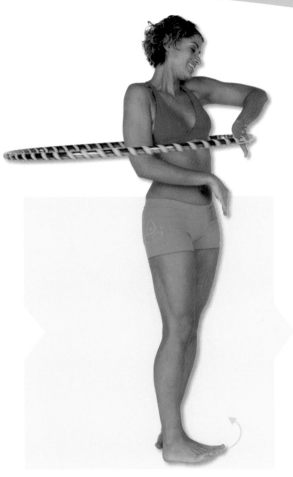

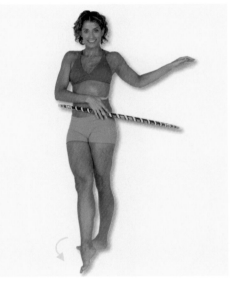

3 Releasing with your WILDWEST hand, let your *shield* hand loosely carry the hoop back down to the level of your waist.

4 When it's at waist level, give the hoop a powerful push into your torso to boomerang it around your waist and resume PUMP.

a tip for triumph

▶ Relax into the flow, knowing that your hands have control of the hoop.

Swish

Use one hand to keep the hoop spinning in front of or alongside your body on a vertical plane. SWISH is a basic building block of many more complex moves.

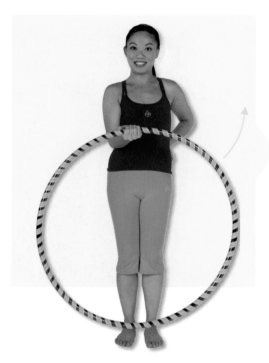

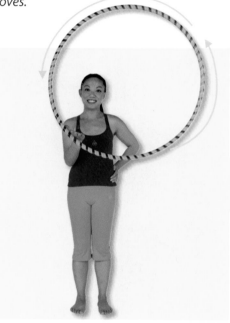

1 Start with the hoop vertically in front of you, holding it on the inside with your palm facing up. Give it a gentle push so it starts revolving with its own momentum.

2 On each rotation, allow the hoop to roll over the back of your hand; briefly grip the hoop to control its angle and speed and send it on to continue its twirl.

NOTE: You should not need to move your shoulder to propel the hoop—instead use the strength of your hand, wrist, and arm.

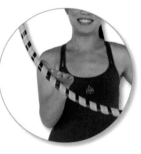

DANCE-IFY IT

Swish can be paired with a simple step-touch to each side. Just don't obstruct the hoop's path by, for example, lifting your knees too high.

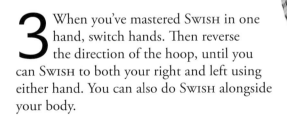

3 When you've mastered Swish in one hand, switch hands. Then reverse the direction of the hoop, until you can Swish to both your right and left using either hand. You can also do Swish alongside your body.

be aware!

▶ If this move causes any discomfort, use both hands with a hand-over-hand turning motion or switch to a lighter hoop.

Nectar

In this simple off-body move, you pass the hoop from hand to hand around your body, keeping it horizontal. Nectar sets up a number of other moves, like the Horizontal Whisper and Pearl.

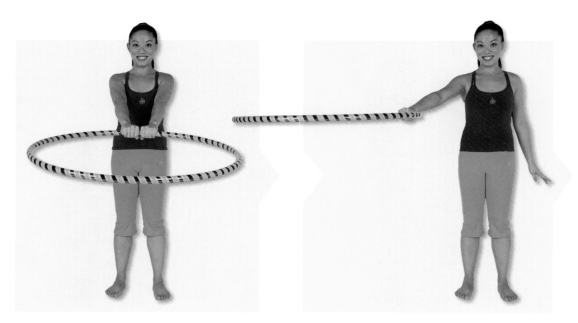

1 Stand holding the hoop on the horizontal in front of you with your right hand gripping on the outside, your palm facing down. If your hoop is too heavy for your wrist, use both hands, thumb to thumb, palms down.

2 Use your right hand to swing the hoop around your body to your right (releasing with the left hand if you were holding it with both hands to start), keeping the hoop horizontal.

be aware!

▶ Hold on tight, or you'll send the hoop hurtling through the air like a giant Frisbee.

DANCE-IFY IT

Play with raising and lowering your body by bending your knees, moving your head side to side and forward and back, or marching in place with your feet.

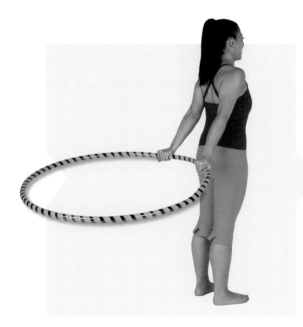

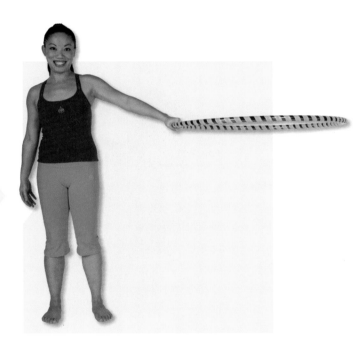

3 As it passes behind you, reach back with your left hand to anticipate and then grab the hoop. Your left hand will be palm down, its pinky facing the pinky of your right hand.

4 With your left hand, continue swinging the hoop around your body, back to the starting position in front. Hand it off to your right hand when they are thumb to thumb and continue from step 2.

• Maintaining the horizontal plane of the hoop is much easier once you gain some speed and momentum. Reverse the flow and do NECTAR counterclockwise as well.

Pearl

Swing the hoop around your neck on the horizontal plane, passing it from hand to hand.
Like a strand of lustrous beads, PEARL is a glamorous move that brings attention to your neck and
face, but it requires patience, practice, and flexible shoulders.

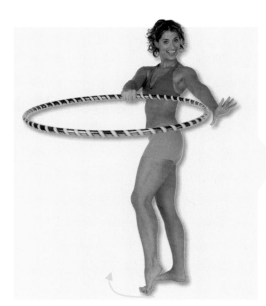

1 Start in NECTAR. To do PEARL you must get some momentum going by passing the hoop from hand to hand, and by turning your body clockwise by taking small steps in the same direction the hoop is moving.

NOTE: These directions are for a clockwise PEARL.

2 When you're ready to do PEARL, the hoop should be in your right hand, with your palm facing the ground. Bring the hoop upward at a slight angle so it can pass just above your left shoulder. Continue turning.

> ### be aware!
> ▶ If you don't turn continuously, you're much more likely
> to get caught in a constricting tangle with this move.

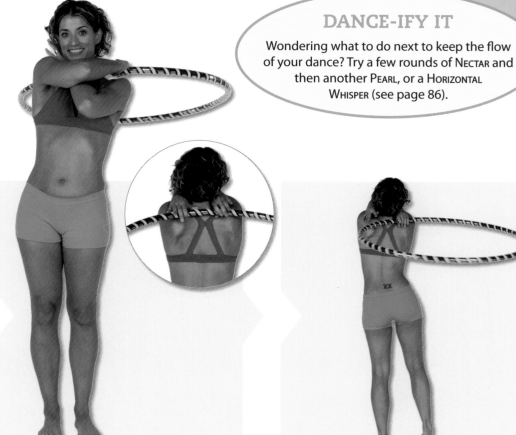

DANCE-IFY IT

Wondering what to do next to keep the flow of your dance? Try a few rounds of NECTAR and then another PEARL, or a HORIZONTAL WHISPER (see page 86).

3 Swing it over the shoulder, reaching your right arm as far as possible to bring the hoop behind your neck. Bring your left hand up to "catch" the hoop as it comes over your right shoulder, crossing forearms in front of your throat. Your left elbow should be *under* your right elbow to bring the hoop farther around.

4 When you've grasped the hoop with your left hand (palm down), release your right hand. As you release, send the hoop off with an extra little push with your fingers. Using your left hand, bring the hoop back into NECTAR.

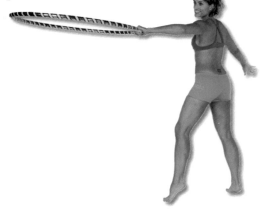

Warrior

In WARRIOR the hoop is swung vertically on alternating sides of the body.

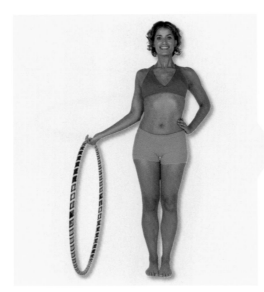

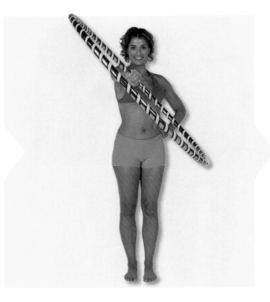

1 Hold the hoop vertically, about a foot out from the right side of your body. It should be hanging loosely in your hand, palm up, and elbow pointing down, as if you were holding a jump rope behind you and were preparing to flip it over your head.

NOTE: These instructions are for right-handed hoopers. Reverse if you're a lefty.

2 Grip the hoop lightly by closing your fingers around it. Lift it back and up, then forward diagonally across the front of your body toward the ground in front of your left foot. The motion in your wrist should feel like you're pouring milk from a pitcher—diagonally across the front of your body.

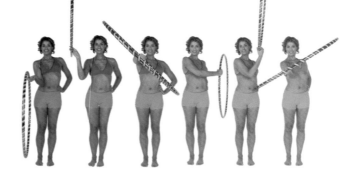

The sequence of movements

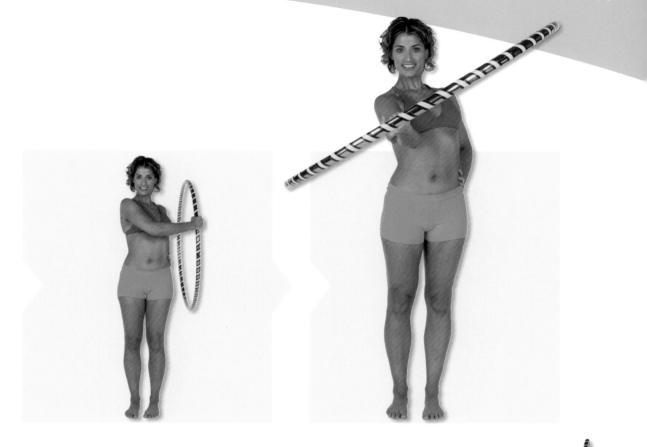

3 Allow the hoop to swing naturally along the side of your body before sending it in the opposite direction.

a tip for triumph

▶ To accomplish WARRIOR, your wrist moves as though you're drawing an infinity symbol in front of you.

4 Without changing your grip but keeping it supple, now flip your wrist as though you're scooping ice cream out of a tub held in your other arm. This should bring your hoop toward the ground in front of your right foot.

• The hoop stays on the vertical plane throughout and as close to the sides of your body as possible. A big hoop may graze the ground, so keep it in the air so that it can swing freely. Your shoulders and torso may swerve rhythmically to stay out of the hoop's path. This is fine.

Toss

Give the hoop a push upward from Swish so the hoop launches into the air on a vertical plane, and catch it as it descends.

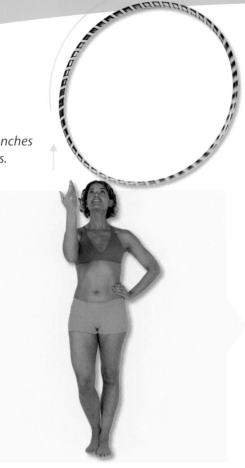

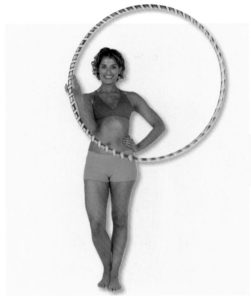

1 Start in Swish in front of you, and then slow it way down while still maintaining the rotation without wobbling.

2 When the hoop rolls from the back of your hand onto the palm, give the hoop a push upward with a flick of your wrist. Release to send the hoop spinning directly up into the air. The hand motion is like the gesture used to ask people to stand up, an assertive, palm-up lift of the hand.

be aware!

▶ Stopping the fall of the hoop with a rigid hand or arm may cause discomfort. Instead, use a supple grip to catch the hoop on the inside as it falls, and follow the hoop's momentum to cushion the contact.

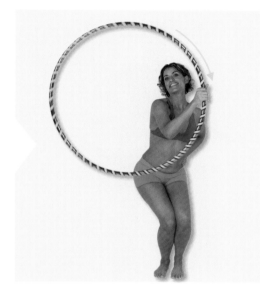

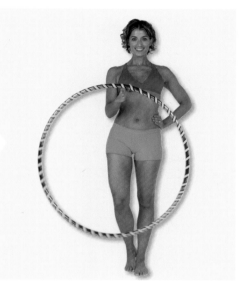

3 Watch the hoop closely so that when it starts to fall you'll be ready to catch it. Extending your hand inside the hoop, grab it and follow its momentum by moving your hand in the same direction as the hoop. (You need to go *with* its movement—like you do when catching a ball.)

4 If your hoop is rotating to the right, you'll be catching the hoop around five o'clock and releasing into Swish just after six. If it's rotating to the left, or counterclockwise, the catch is at about seven, and the release at about six. Now push and release the hoop into Swish again.

• Until you get comfortable, keep the toss low and controlled. You shouldn't have to take more than one step in order to catch it. After you've mastered the catch, you can send it higher and higher, as your overhead space allows.

Slinky

In SLINKY, your hands alternate, darting down into the space between your hoop and your body, as you keep the hoop orbiting your waist in PUMP.

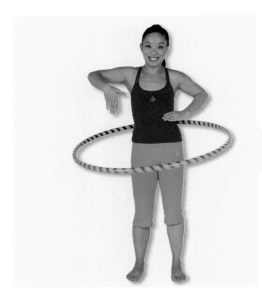

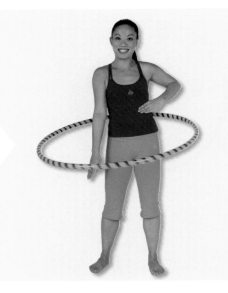

1 Start in PUMP. As the hoop circles your waist, notice when and where you see an opening between the hoop and your body.

2 Once you've got a handle on the rhythm, dart a hand into that open space, shooting your fingers straight down and then *immediately* back out before the hoop rolls over your hand.

a tip for triumph

▶ You need to really *feel* your way into this move. To develop this kinesthetic awareness, experiment with your eyes closed and learn to rely on the sensation of the hoop pressing against one side of your body to tell you that a space is opening up on the opposite side for SLINKY.

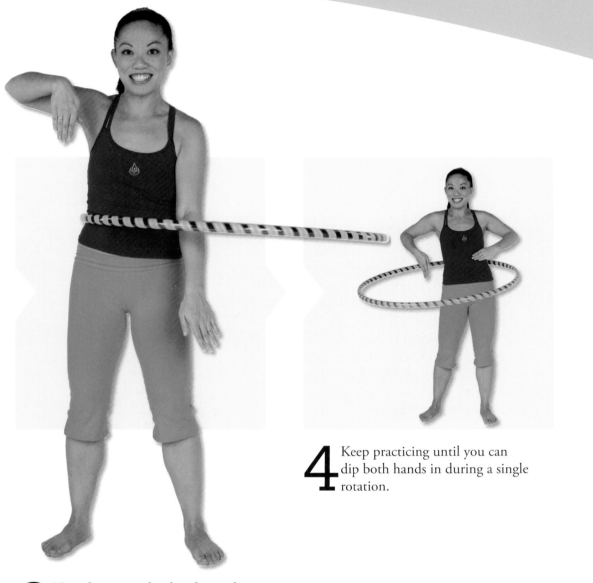

4 Keep practicing until you can dip both hands in during a single rotation.

3 Now dip your other hand into the open space. Extend your arm as far as possible.

A Flowering Bud

I WAS AN ONLY CHILD, AND MY FAMILY MOVED almost every year when I was growing up so I was always the "new girl" in school. I quickly learned that life at a new school was easier if I wasn't noticed. I remember sitting with my shoulders hunched forward and my arms tucked tightly into my lap to take up as little space as possible. It was my protective stance. I was a nail-biter, and sometimes I'd hide my hands between my thighs out of shame.

When I was fifteen years old, I started working in restaurants, and I did that off and on for twelve years. At the end of the day, my feet hurt and the rest of my body felt almost numb. I was still inhibited, and in personal interactions I felt myself holding back what I had to offer, my hands restless and fidgety.

My body finally found the freedom to express itself when I started doing Nia years later. I gained strength, flexibility, and most of all, grace. I learned to stand tall and proudly take up space in the world. And I used my hands freely to express myself. Then when I discovered the hoop, I blossomed— literally, it felt like I was the center of a flower, and my newly liberated arms were petals.

Unrestrained, free-flowing dance brought me into my body. But what was special about the hoop was that I had to learn to be in a relationship with an object while I moved. The hoop's got its own groove. I have to move in rhythm with it, knowing when to yield, when to anticipate it, and when to respond.

And the hoop helped free more than my body. It freed me to help others. Once the new girl afraid to take up space or use her voice, I am now a life coach empowering others to use theirs. Sometimes I invite a client into the hoop to offer her a safe container to express herself. And as soon as she learns her first move, usually the first thing she'll do is lift her arms up high above her head with a squeal of delight. And I can't help but smile and say "Yes!"

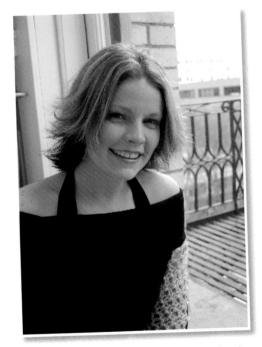

Name: Candice
Occupation: Life Coach

Mind Over Motion

I encourage students to learn how subtle shifts in the positions of their fingers, hands, and elbows feel different. Wondering what on earth I mean? Try this: While in PUMP, hold your palms face-up. Note how it feels. Then turn your hands over so your palms face the floor. Can you perceive a change? For most people, palms-up is energizing and uplifting, while palms-down is grounding and calming. Experiment with the different sensations created by moving each of your joints in a variety of dimensions and directions.

Adding visualization and your imagination to any movement can deepen the experience. For example, you can pretend to push something heavy, to swirl your hands in water, or to shoot lasers through your fingertips. Holding these kinds of images in your mind in order to add purpose and texture to a movement is a concept called *ideokinesis*. Because it links your imagination to your physical body, ideokinesis improves coordination between your muscles and nervous system. Images naturally prompt you to explore the space around you more fully, in multiple dimensions.

Andre Bernard, a major contributor to the field of ideokinesis, notes that the image "needs to make a strong impression on the nervous system and to do that it has to be unusual . . . by being outrageous, ridiculous, or beautiful, or anything that is excessive." In HoopGirl classes and in this book I use a lot of vivid, strong images to deepen the experience for your body and your mind.

The Matrix

IMAGINE YOU ARE A CHARACTER FROM the movie *The Matrix* and have the ability to torque and bend your torso in any direction, while you are hooping in PUMP. Lean your head and torso all the way to one side while keeping your hoop spinning, and then the other. Surprise yourself with your supernatural abilities.

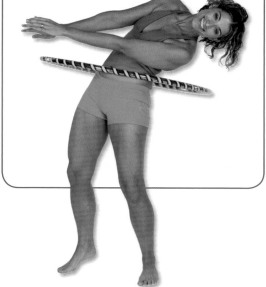

THE MOVES

Just Legs

LUNGES, LIFTS & LEAPS
TO SCULPT YOUR LOWER BODY

The secret to achieving your ideal lower body isn't really such a secret. The key is to combine a healthy diet (see Nutritional Notes on page 203) and cardiovascular exercise to reduce excess fat all over your body with strength and resistance training that focuses on the muscles of your buns, thighs, and calves. Cardio and resistance work go hand in hand (or in this case, leg in leg) because building muscles increases metabolism which means you'll burn more calories during cardio workouts. It's a delicious cycle.

As we've seen, hooping has cardio covered. Energetic hooping can burn over six hundred calories per hour, raising your heart rate and deepening your breathing, so that the oxygen in your blood flows to your muscles. As for strength-building and toning, the weight of the hoop plus that of your own body create the resistance that builds leaner and stronger muscles. The approximately one-and-a-half-pound weight of a hoop may not seem like much, but at about a hundred rotations per minute, you're going to feel your muscles exerting themselves—trust me.

This chapter will focus on specific leg movements, but remember that all the core hooping moves work the legs as well. For example, in PUMP, your legs have to push into the ground to power the movements of your hips and keep you stabilized.

Grace Anatomy

Before getting moving, let's scan some key features of your lower body landscape that play important roles in hoopdancing.

Knees. As the body's largest joint, the knees allow us to bend and raise our bodies. They can carry our entire weight. By bending the knees, we relieve pressure on the lower back. The angle created by the knees determines the position of the pelvis and affects posture. Knees launch you into the air and then help absorb the impact of landing. Awareness of all these connections helps hoopers bend their knees with purpose.

Ankles. These little guys allow multi-dimensional movement. They are the key to pivoting and turning inside the hoop. Don't take their gifts for granted! Constantly pivoting on only one foot in one direction can cause injury. Allow your ankles to teach you the value of switching directions. Regularly give your dominant ankle a break and build strength in the other side. For turns and pivots on hard flooring, smooth-soled dance sneakers can make the ride much easier on your ankles, unlike street sneakers, which stick like suction cups to the ground.

Feet. Toes are the fingers of the feet. Skilled toes can splay, grab, and even snap! Pay attention to how you step and notice which part of your foot you are favoring: which side? The ball? The toes? The heel? Are you flattening or curving the arch? After a jump, make sure to land on the balls of your feet, allowing them and the calves to absorb the impact gradually. Hooping uses the feet and toes not only for balance but for expression. For example, think of pointing your toes versus flexing your foot. Try barefoot hooping for a blissful romp through childhood memories.

Strong Not Skinny

There is more to the story of your legs than just getting lean and looking pretty. Legs and feet connect you to the earth. They allow you to *ground,* or to release excess energy, to focus, and to gain stability and power from the surface that supports you. Your legs not only move you forward, but can also change your direction; on a symbolic level, they move you through life. Do you feel stable or tentative, agile or awkward? To focus on the legs is to examine not only where you are headed but also how you get there.

Hooping helps you redefine the beauty of your legs in terms of *power, poise,* and *stamina*. Think of a cheetah running at seventy-five miles per hour over a savanna, or picture the furious footwork of a flamenco dancer. Strong—as opposed to skinny—is where it's at. Powerful legs translate into a precise, articulate, and energized way of hooping, dancing . . . and moving through the world.

This is especially important when contemplating your thighs—this habitually criticized, judged, and unloved terrain of the female body. Let's face it—for most women, the media's images of slender, airbrushed legs are unattainable. And still we buy into them.

Hooping brings opportunities to feel grateful for your legs. While you groove, gyrate, and crouch, you'll appreciate their energy, stability, and reliability. Not only do they sustain you in Limbo and activate as you do Whisper, but they support you everywhere you go and no matter what you decide to do in life.

hold in
THIG H ESTEEM

Start making it a habit to reflect on what is good about your legs. While breathing deeply, say each phrase aloud, allowing yourself to really feel its truth. It may be helpful to look in a mirror as you do this.

★ *I love my legs exactly as they are!*

★ *My legs are my friends. I accept and take care of my friends.*

★ *Every day my legs become more gorgeous.*

★ *My calves are strong and beautiful.*

★ *I enjoy nurturing my legs with baths, massage, and pedicures.*

Fancy Footwork

Your feet and legs have unlimited dance potential. For hoopers wanting to add more spice to their leg and foot movements, the many genres of dance provide a vast menu to choose from. You can employ the footwork from any other dance form while doing Pump. Urban street dance like hip-hop, Pop and Lock, Krumping, and B-Girl styles provide percussive steps that can be syncopated with hoop rotations. From belly dance and Bollywood dancing you can borrow flowing movements, and from martial arts, powerful, linear steps and

Legs-ercises

LET'S START YOUR LEGWORK BY ADDING THREE common exercises to a couple of upper body moves you learned in the last chapter. Although these moves are probably familiar to you, correct form really enhances the impact on your muscles and is key to preventing injuries.

LUNGES

1 While keeping the hoop above your head in WILDWEST, let's lunge! Lunges are great for your glutes (your rear) and your quads (the front part of your thighs).

2 Start with your feet shoulder-width apart (to gauge that distance, place both fists between your feet) and your weight equally distributed. With your right hand doing WILDWEST, step directly forward (not inward toward the centerline of your body) with the right foot. Keeping your back straight, bend your right knee to lower your torso toward the ground. Your knee should line up with your hip and ankle, and never extend in front of your ankle. You should not feel a strain in your hips.

3 Come back to standing, switch the WILDWEST to your left hand, and lunge with the left leg. The lower to the ground you lunge, the more powerfully you will have to engage your glutes and quad to return to standing. Alternate legs and keep switching hands to WILDWEST. Do about eight on each side.

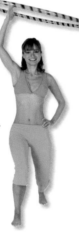

SQUATS

1 Squats are great for working all the major muscles below your waist. Keep your weight on your heels to really work your hamstrings (the backs of your thighs).

2 With your legs shoulder-width apart and your weight evenly balanced, swing the hoop in WILDWEST. Press your belly button in toward your spine to tighten your abs. Without lifting your heels off the ground, inhale as you lower your body back and down as low as you can go. Pretend you are sitting down in a chair. Then, tighten your butt and thigh muscles and exhale as you slowly stand back up. Do two sets of eight, switching hands and changing the direction of the hoop after the first set.

HEEL RAISES

1 Let your hoop rest in front of you on the ground, with your hands resting lightly on it. Now let's do some Heel Raises. Your calf muscles will adore you.

2 Stand with your feet directly under your hips. Exhale as you rise up on the balls of your feet, lifting your heels off the ground. Hold for a count of 10, pressing into the ground with distinct awareness of your big toes. Inhale and lower your heels down, slowly. Repeat ten times.

kicks. You can adapt ballroom styles like the fox trot or waltz, or the more flamboyant Latin dances to lend dynamism and drama.

To inspire you to create your own unique fusion, let's do PUMP and add one Latin and one ballroom step. Patterns of footwork like these shift your weight and affect the position of your hips, so they might knock your hoop out of orbit. Embrace the challenge.

SALSA

Step forward with one foot, shift your weight back to the other (the central leg), and then bring the forward foot back so both are back together at the starting point. Hold for a count. Next, step back with the leg that was stationary at the start, shift your weight forward to the central leg, and then step forward with the traveling leg so your feet are side by side again. Pause.

GRAPEVINE

To do the Grapevine to the right: 1) Step to the side with your right foot, then 2) step across in front of it with your left foot. 3) Take another step to the side with your right foot, and 4) step behind it with the left. 5) Take another step to the right. 6) Bring your left foot next to it. Repeat the sequence as far to the right as you want to go. Do the same sequence to the left.

hop-to-it PLAYLIST

High energy house music to get your groove on.

#	Song	Artist
1.	PETALPUSHING	Miguel Migs
2.	LADADI (DADA)	Davison Ospina
3.	LOVE AND HAPPINESS	River Ocean
4.	CALABRIA 2007 (Club Mix)	Enur
5.	RAIN DOWN LOVE (2007 Club Mix)	Freemasons (ft. Siedah Garrett)
6.	LOVE WILL FIND A WAY (Secret Soul Remix)	Cambis & Freakquence Lab (ft. Kwame Remy)
7.	GOOD NIGHT	Brown Sugar, Niko De Luka (ft. Dawn Tallman-Romain Curtis Remix)
8.	YOU ARE MY HOUSE	Oscar P. (ft. Ama- Original Mix)
9.	I LIKE THE WAY YOU MOVE (Radio Mix)	Ariano Kina
10.	SHINE ON (Radio Mix)	R.I.O.

Horizontal Whisper

While passing the hoop around your body on the horizontal plane, lift one leg to the side and pass the hoop under it, from one hand to the other.

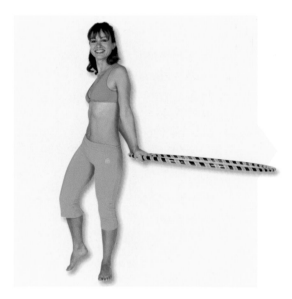

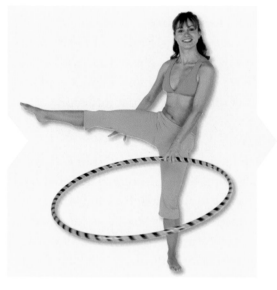

1 Start in NECTAR (page 68) allowing the hoop to get some momentum moving on a horizontal plane around your body.

2 Engage your abs, pulling your belly button toward your spine, and lift the leg on the opposite side of your body from the hoop. Extend the leg straight out to the side as high as you can, and point your toes. Really press into the ground with your standing foot to stabilize and balance.

vocalize

▶ Experiment with saying "Whisper" in a soft voice, as the hoop passes below your leg, emphasizing the "sss" to remind you to relax and breathe. Then try shouting "ha!" as you kick your leg up. Just as in martial arts, creating this sound allows powerful abdominal contraction. Switch back and forth between the soft and loud sounds and notice how it affects your form.

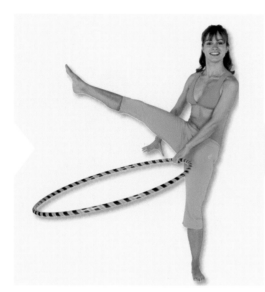

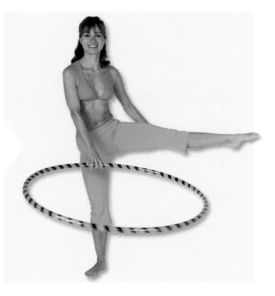

3 Pass the hoop under the raised leg (a few inches below it), releasing it to the opposite hand as you do so. While under the raised thigh, your hands should stay a whisper's distance from your supporting leg. Keep your head high, your shoulders back and down, and your chest open. Lower the leg as soon as the hoop has passed underneath.

4 Continue in NECTAR. When you're ready, as the hoop is coming in front of you, raise your other leg, point it straight out in front of you, and pass the hoop under it.

• You can WHISPER (raise a leg) each time the hoop comes around in front of you, or you can do a few rounds of NECTAR in between each WHISPER. Alternate which leg you lift each time.

Vertical Whisper

While Swishing the hoop in front of you, lift up one leg and pass the hoop under your thigh, from hand to hand.

NOTE: Before doing this move, test the size of your hoop by standing it on the ground and swinging a leg over. If you can't, you need a smaller hoop for this move.

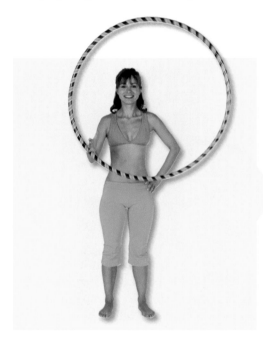

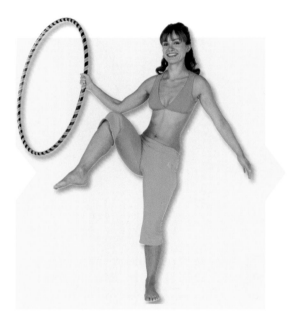

1 Start the hoop in Swish (page 66) in front of your body.

2 As the hoop swoops toward the ground on its downward trajectory, engage your abs and lift one knee high. (It doesn't matter which knee.) You can extend your leg straight or keep the knee bent with your foot pointed.

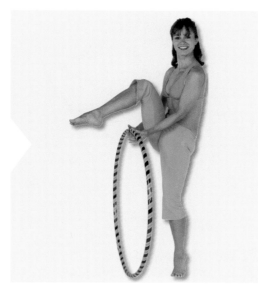

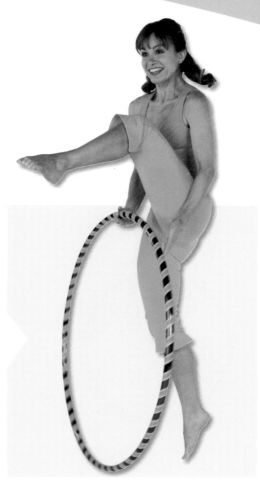

3 With your hand on the inside of the hoop, palm facing up, pass the hoop underneath the raised leg to the opposite hand. The hands should face pinky-to-pinky before you release with the SWISH hand. Resume SWISH.

4 When you're ready to WHISPER again, use the opposite leg. Alternate legs to give both sides an equal workout. Jump up in the moment of the pass for an added thrill.

Step

Transition from off-body to on-body by bringing the hoop around in your hand, lowering it, and stepping into it. STEP provides a smooth transition back to PUMP.

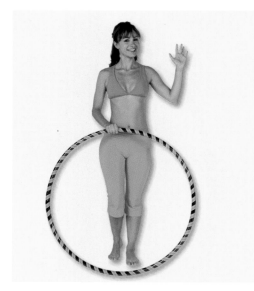

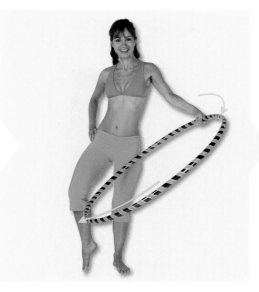

1 Identify the hand opposite of how your hoop travels in INFLOW. (For example, if your hoop usually rotates to your right, use your left hand.)

2 Bring the hoop in front of you in your INFLOW direction and tilt it so it slopes to the ground.

challenge yourself

▶ Once you've mastered STEP, take it to the next level with BOUNCE. This time, as you tilt the hoop to the ground, launch off both feet simultaneously and *jump* inside the hoop at its lowest point. Continue as with STEP. If BOUNCE is too adventurous for your knees, ankles, or feet, stick with STEP. You know your body best.

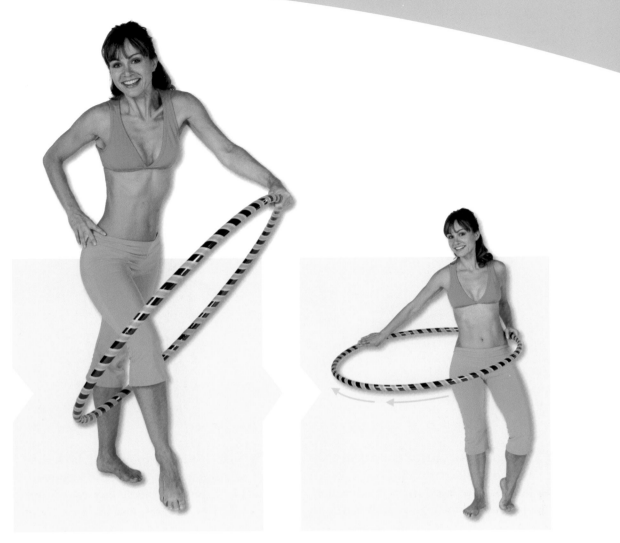

3 Step inside the hoop with the foot that's opposite the hand holding the hoop. Then quickly step in with your other foot.

Keep taking steps to turn your body in the direction the hoop is moving.

4 When both feet are inside the hoop, immediately push the hoop out to the side with the opposite hand and launch into PUMP. Boomerang it!

Skip

Take the hoop off your core by grasping the hoop in your hand and stepping out of it.

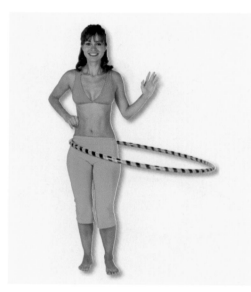

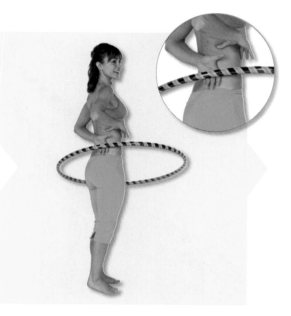

1 Begin in PUMP (page 20). Identify the hand opposite of the direction your hoop is traveling. Turn in the direction the hoop is rotating by taking small steps with your feet.

2 Slide that hand around your back as far as possible, so it rests near the opposite hip. Your palm should face away from your body, your fingers pointing down. (This is the same position as in FLOAT, page 60.)

challenge yourself

▶ Once you've mastered SKIP, you can jump out with both feet at once. In SPRING, as you tilt the hoop toward the ground, bend your knees to spring-load your legs and jump over the lowest point of the hoop with both feet simultaneously. Land outside the hoop, switch the grip of your hand, and go from there! If SPRING is too bold for your joints, remember the Pleasure Principle, and stick with the SKIP.

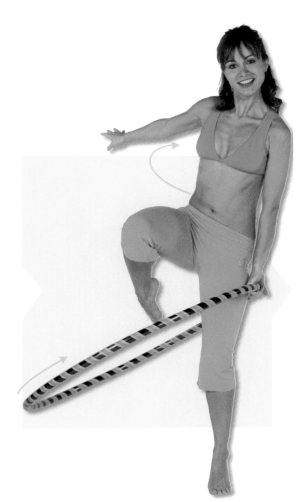

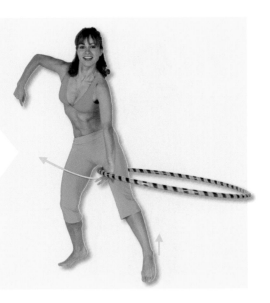

3 Slow your PUMP down as far as you can without letting the hoop drop. As it rolls over your palm, grasp the hoop and bring it around to the front of your body. Tilt it so it slopes to the ground, away from the hand holding the hoop. Prepare to step out with the foot opposite that hand.

4 Step out of the hoop with one foot, then quickly follow with the other. Allow the hoop to roll over the back of your hand and then into your palm before gripping it again. You'll end with your palm facing the ground, as in NECTAR.

Leap

During WARRIOR, dart through the hoop, channeling your inner gazelle. The plane of the hoop should stay as close to vertical as possible.

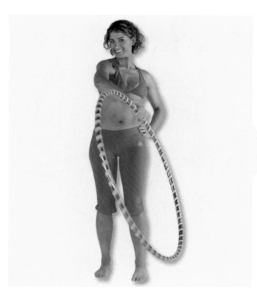

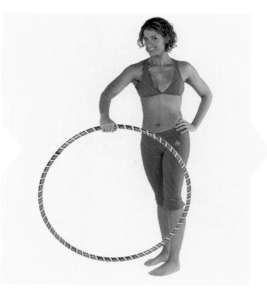

1 Start in WARRIOR (page 72), bringing the hoop across your body with the "pouring" wrist.

2 Then turn the hoop slightly by twisting your wrist so your knuckles turn toward the ground. This should bring the hoop in front of you on an angle with an open area to spring into, almost like a jump rope.

a tip for triumph

▶ Allow the momentum of the hoop to help you swing it up behind you, keeping the grip supple. If you are swinging the hoop too slowly, it will take more wrist strength to flip the hoop. To assist the flip, bring your other hand onto the hoop after you've leapt, releasing it once you're back in the "pouring" position of WARRIOR.

DANCE-IFY IT

Experiment with placing your other hand on your hip. For a dazzling display of athleticism, do multiple consecutive Leaps.

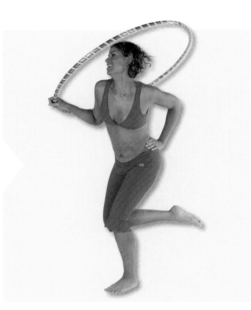

3 Hop into the hoop, leading with the foot opposite the hand holding the hoop. As soon as you have leapt through it, swivel the hoop in your grip so it flips up behind you, over your head, and down along your side. The motion of your wrist is like turning a car key in the ignition.

4 The hoop should wind up back in the pre-leap or "pouring" position of Warrior. Avoid flipping your hoop too far over. It should only swivel enough to continue in Warrior. With practice, you'll be able to jump through the hoop with both feet at the same time.

Dolphin

Leap straight forward through the vertically held hoop. The key to the illusion is keeping the hoop moving on a completely vertical plane in front of you.

NOTE: Before diving in, let's walk through the move in slow motion here.

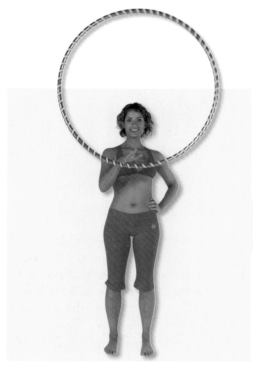

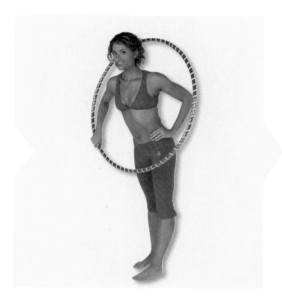

1 Start in SWISH (page 66) with the hoop spinning directly in front of you. If you're right-handed, the hoop should be in your right hand, SWISHING the hoop so that it turns counterclockwise.

2 Immediately after the hoop rolls over the back of your hand onto your palm, grip the hoop on the inside and lean your upper body inside the hoop, as though you're leaning through a window. (You may need to duck your head slightly.) As you do this, swivel the hoop a little so your grip shifts toward the outside.

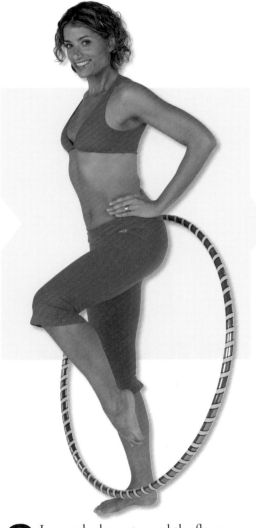

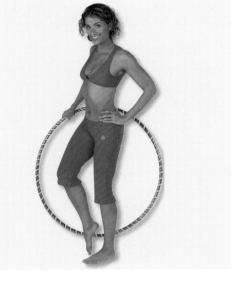

4 Step through the opening with your left and then your right foot, continuing to swivel the hoop in your grip so it is comfortable. The hoop is now on a vertical plane behind you, about hip height, with your palm facing down. Allow it to roll over the back of your hand as you bring it in front of your body and continue in SWISH.

3 Lower the hoop toward the floor creating a window for your feet to step through.

5 Now speed up the move so that the hoop is in continual motion in your right hand, and you are jumping straight through it.

visualize

▶ Imagine yourself as the trainer who dramatically raises the ring above the water for the dolphin to jump through. Now imagine yourself as the supple dolphin gracefully arching through the ring to wild applause. DOLPHIN embodies both these roles.

From Injury to Victory

TEN YEARS AGO I WAS IN A CAR ACCIDENT that injured my lower back at my sacrum. Before the accident I weighed 128 pounds. I'd always been fit from doing lots of different activities, including regular running and weight lifting. But after the accident I was unable to sleep, bend, sit, or twist without pain. In the years it took to recover, I reached 195 pounds and 60 percent fat. I couldn't believe it: I was only thirty-three years old!

It was a vicious circle: Whenever I tried to exercise I just hurt myself all over again. I felt like I was spiraling downward. I felt unattractive. I was depressed. I wasn't the only one who noticed my unhappy transformation, either—my boyfriends and my mom kept voicing their concerns about my health.

About this time I heard about hooping classes. I had no idea how great an aerobic workout it would be. After the first fifteen minutes, I was sweating and out of breath . . . and even though I felt like a total dork doing the moves, I was having a blast. By the second class, the moves were already starting to come more naturally, like magic! By the third class, I was totally hooked.

I decided to start taking this hooping seriously (funny, right?), using it to replace the running I had done before. Unlike running, hooping is a low-impact aerobic exercise, so it doesn't strain my knees. I also resumed weight lifting—very carefully. The new regime (hooping and weight lifting) has cut my body fat percentage by a third! And I'm definitely more toned.

Amazingly, after ten years of chronic back pain due to the accident, I'm currently pain-free! I can only assume this is from the hooping because it's the only thing I've done differently.

Plus, because hooping's so fun, in addition to my scheduled workouts, I usually hoop another couple of hours a week with friends!

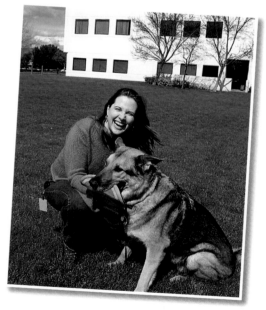

Name: Stephanie
Occupation: Technical Support Engineer

Freedom of Expression

LIBERATE YOUR LEGS (AND OTHER LIMBS) BY focusing on one of the following ideas as you hoop. Explore and fill the space around you, giving your movements the textures that each image calls for. Let your muscles engage with a strong new purpose— you haven't stalked any prey while hooping before, have you? Feel free to improvise and conjure up other images to inspire you as well.

seaweed tide ▶ loose, flowing, ecstatic

Imagine that your legs, torso, arms, and neck are strands of seaweed, tumbling through the ocean waves. Undulate in organic patterns. Let your legs be carried by the currents. Let each finger become a separate strand, floating on the waves and dancing through the salty water.

bubble play ▶ gentle, light, delicate

Envision yourself surrounded by giant transparent bubbles. Delicately catch them so they don't burst, then blow them aloft again. Tenderly bounce them off your feet, knees, elbows, and head. Twirl one like a basketball on the tip of one extended finger.

diamond gown ▶ luxurious, sparkling, delightful

Imagine you are a regal empress with strings of diamonds dangling from your waist. Dance and twirl through the castle ballroom, feeling the weight of the precious stones as they sway. Run your fingers through the glittering strands as you do SLINKY.

jungle hunt ▶ lithe, focused, primal

Become a stealthy tiger stalking its prey. Press your limbs against your core to camouflage yourself in the jungle. Spring-load your legs and ready your shoulders for the pounce. Bat a mosquito away with a heavy paw. Twitch your tail and bare your teeth.

honey pot ▶ slow, warm, sensual

Imagine that your hoop is full of golden honey. Stir the thick sweetness with your arms. Move your feet and legs against the stickiness. Dip your fingers in and taste the nectar. Tip the hoop from side to side and let the honey drip over.

THE MOVES

6

Getting in Flow

FUSE MOVES
& CREATE DANCE

Maybe this is your routine: Three times a week, PUMP during the morning show, switching to PULSE during every commercial break. Then ten HORIZONTAL WHISPERS with the left leg, ten with the right. Twenty VERTICAL WHISPERS—ten on each side. Twenty slo-mo biceps-burning WARRIORS. NECTAR for ten rounds to the right, then ten rounds to the left—while marching in place. Cool down with a slow PUMP for two minutes and stretch.

Good for you! You're tending to a lot of key muscles in your core, legs, and arms all while taking in the morning news. You're a multitasker to boot!

Of course, you're welcome to take this approach to hooping. It's the way you probably learned other forms of fitness: sustained cardio activity paired with reps of resistance training to build strength in specific muscle groups. You will certainly see physical results by committing to this kind of hooping practice.

But if you're like the thousands of people who get bored with repetition and avoid the gym at all costs, turning hooping into hoopdance may suit you better.

Hoopdancing offers a mindblowing, infinite number of ways in which you can connect the three ingredients of music, body, and hoop. It's this vast possibility that makes hoopdancing so addictive. Hoopers fall asleep at night envisioning new ways to link moves, and they wake up eager to enact the routine they dreamed up while asleep. While stuck behind their desks, they fantasize about transitioning from SWISH to VERTICAL WHISPER to DOLPHIN to WARRIOR to LEAP to SWISH to TOSS. Can it be done? With practice? They can't wait to try it at home. Some of them even have hoops on hand at the office, for quick hoop-relief in the middle of an otherwise hectic day. Flowing moves together or making up a routine isn't about becoming a performer. It is about deepening the fun, challenge, and interest of your hooping sessions. It's about keeping it fresh! It's also about giving the neurological circuits that connect your brain and your muscles a workout, as you translate ideas in your head into a complex series of movements, also known as *dance*.

Dance, How?

In class, I like to say that teaching hooping without dancing is like teaching soccer without running. Yet how, exactly, does one dance, let alone with a hoop?

To dance is to listen with your whole body. You have to start by finding the beat, which sets the tempo like a metronome. Have you ever stood next to a big speaker at a nightclub? The beat is the steady pounding that vibrates your body to the core. If getting your body moving with the beat doesn't come naturally, try this:

Count out loud every time you hear the most prominent beats. Feel the sound resonate in your bones. Start tapping a foot to your count. Then start lifting your knees to it. Let the sound come into your chest and pulsate your torso to it. Alternate lifting each arm out to the side with it, then forward and back. Turn your head left and right to it. See if you can get every part of your body—fingers, hands, wrists, elbows, shoulders, torso, head, hips, knees, and feet—connected to the beat.

Now you need to add another element to the equation—your hoop! So while still counting along with and tapping a foot to the beat, grab your hoop and launch into Pump. Speed up or slow your hoop so that you feel it bumping your body at the same time you feel—and call out—the beat. **This is the fundamental experience of rhythm in hooping—when the hoop plays your body like a drum, in sync with the music.**

Usually, there's also a melody that sails along the top of the beat. To respond to the melody, let your limbs and head be swept along. Use your body like a giant paintbrush to express the emotions behind the lyrics. For example, if you are dancing to Middle Eastern melodies, you could move your arms in undulating waves.

The final challenge is to respond to both the beat and melody simultaneously. An easy way to do this is to keep your feet, knees, and torso pulsating to the beat. Once these parts are locked into the rhythm, allow your arms and head to begin swaying to the melody and

deeper meanings
OF DANCE

The urge to dance is ancient and innate. For over nine thousand years, humans have moved their bodies to tell stories, to express emotions, to heal, to commune with the divine, and to punctuate important moments in life—harvests, the changing of seasons, deaths, and births. From a very young age, babies wiggle and shimmy as they discover their bodies. Children bounce instinctively to melody and rhythm. We dance at weddings. We dance with the people we love. We dance to celebrate.

Iris Stewart, author of *Sacred Woman, Sacred Dance,* suggests that dance can become a ritual of self-discovery and can awaken a sense of spirituality: "Every dancer knows her goal is to get to that point where the body no longer stands in the way but becomes the instrument of the soul's expression." In a time when we have fewer rites of passage, healing ceremonies, or universally shared spiritual traditions, dancing can be a channel through which we connect to the sacred.

moving through the space around you three-dimensionally. If the hoop is on your core, it follows the beat. When the hoop is off-body, in your hands, it will probably follow the melody.

While first exploring hoopdancing, stay in Pump. This will give you maximum freedom of movement. As you feel more comfortable connecting the beat and the melody to your body and hoop, experiment with other moves, such as Slinky and Booty Blitz. You'll find that some moves, like Leap and Dolphin, are so all-encompassing that

feel the
MUSIC

The vibrations that translate to your ear as music have profound physiological effects—they impact your blood pressure, respiration, and pulse. In your brain, they cause a storm of electrical activity. Synapses fire. Memories and images can be evoked, and breathtaking emotions can wash over you . . . Let these infuse your dance as well.

Sampling different kinds of music can have surprising consequences for your dance. Maybe you dislike a song included in one of the playlists here. I encourage you to stick with it for a while. New music can inspire you to move in different ways. Free yourself of the need to "like" the music. Instead, just *feel* the music, no matter what. Let each instrument and its emotional quality resonate inside you, and then embody it or answer it. You'll develop the ability to *respond* instead of *react*.

there is little "space" to dance simultaneously. Hoopdancers use these kinds of complex moves to bookend or punctuate their ongoing dance.

With time and practice, the beats and the melody will overtake you and your hoop. You'll lose yourself in the sensations, and all three partners—music, body, hoop—will be in sync. That's what's meant by achieving "flow" in hoopdance.

Transition and Flow

OK, OK, I'm dancing already, I'm dancing, you say. But how do I know which move to do next, and how do I move gracefully from one move to another? String moves together? Which one should I do next?

There's magic in combinations. Like the instant in a foreign language class when you compose your first sentence from the basic vocabulary you've acquired, or a one-of-a-kind necklace you string from a grab bag of beads. In hooping, we all start with similar components—the moves—yet the way each of us combines them and adds our own flourishes makes them uniquely our own. Read through the suggestions below on how to arrange moves, but remember to stay open to the magic that simply unfolds as you dance.

FLOW POINTERS

1. If the hoop is on your core (for example PUMP), you can either do another kind of core move (such as BOOTY BLITZ, SLINKY, or LIMBO) or use a move that transitions the hoop to off-body (for example, FLOAT or SKIP).

2. If the hoop is off-body, which plane is it on? It's easiest to transition between two moves in the same plane. For example, while the hoop is vertical for SWISH, you can easily move into VERTICAL WHISPER or DOLPHIN or WARRIOR. If the hoop is horizontal in NECTAR, you can transition smoothly to WILDWEST, PEARL, or HORIZONTAL WHISPER . . . or you could do a STEP to get back inside the hoop for some core moves.

3. If you want to switch between horizontal and vertical planes while still dancing, punctuate the change with a pause and a corresponding moment in the music. For example, from SWISH, allow the hoop to slip through your hands so it drops to the ground on the vertical. Allow it to stand on the ground for a couple of beats while you use your feet (stomp), knees (squat), hands

(tap on the top of the hoop), and/or head (bop side to side) to dance, accentuating the transition. Then grab the hoop and swing it into NECTAR, a basic horizontal position.

4. Practice, practice, practice! As you get comfortable with a variety of moves, spontaneous combinations will effortlessly emerge.

> "Stepping into Flow with my hoop is akin to entering a powerful river of Energy, one that is fast-moving and washes away the moment-to-moment experience of Self, replacing it with an experience of Source."
>
> — *Spiral*

With time, you'll get to a point where things simply fall into place, and one move flows into the next. There is no thinking, only breathing, feeling, and following your intuition. You know flow when you feel it—gliding along, graceful, easy, and effortless.

Allowing Flow

YEARS AGO, I'D HEARD ABOUT THE YOGIC PATH as a way to "be here now" and to open oneself to life's synchronicities. Those concepts felt so off-limits. They didn't fit with the rational world I knew. Instead, I plugged away at a nine-to-five job that was focused on material gain, and I was mired in fear and extreme forward thinking—nowhere near the now. I didn't *feel*, I *thought*. But I wanted to be different. I wanted to allow myself to live on the ebb and flow of life's ocean.

I've been in the hoop now for three years, practicing yoga for eight—not that I can tell where one ends and the other begins. I guess you could say it was through yoga that I found the hoop, but I think of it more as getting permission: Yoga gave me permission to come into the flow of hoopdance because of how it invited me into my Self and into my body.

I felt soft in the hoop's circle, impressionable. I don't know if it was the symbolic resonance (the circle as eternity or wholeness) or the constant physical contact—but I stopped *thinking* and started *experiencing*. Suddenly, everything I had heard for years in yoga became clear. The veils lifted. Inside the hoop I became totally present in the moment. I reunited with a deeper Self. And with each breath I was reminded of what it means to be connected with something larger than myself. An expansive shift occurred.

This "flow" with the hoop is my meditation—an act of moving in a steady, continuous stream, in harmony with my breath. The experience of flow rendered me capable of accepting any situation.

A white flag. A surrendering of the need to "do" and instead just *allow*. Through the hoop, I've learned that *allowing*—going with the flow instead of fighting against the current—reveals a purpose, a "coming into self" with no room for apology. This higher purpose is what the world needs. Because what are we here for if not to live to our highest potential, if not to live by the creed of our own unique and innate gifts?

When I hoop, I hold that knowledge in my heart and move from it. I send my purpose out, whirling and spiraling it into existence. Breathe. Release. Expand. Dream. Breathe.

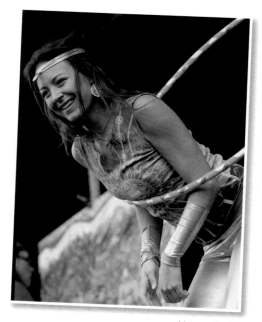

Name: Shakti
Occupation: Copywriter

Transcendent Flow

Hooping in flow provides a sense of immediacy and centeredness, similar to what athletes call being "in the Zone." True flow connects you with an inner point of stillness. It feels like letting go and arriving all at once. You can stop *trying* as there is nothing to achieve. It has elements of surrender and moments of direction, but at all times there is a feeling of oneness between the hoop and your body.

In his book *Flow,* psychologist Mihaly Csikszentmihalyi describes flow as an optimal state of being: "People typically feel strong, alert, in effortless control, unselfconscious, and at the peak of their abilities. Both the sense of time and emotional problems seem to disappear, and there is an exhilarating feeling of transcendence."

If you aren't feeling "in flow," you can help access this state by consciously centering yourself while hooping. Allow your breathing to remind you to "be here now." You can create a mantra by saying "in" during an extended inhalation, and "out" during a long exhalation.

the fluid mix
PLAYLIST

Spirit-infused sounds for meditative movement

1.	BREATHE	Blue Stone
2.	HARE KRISHNA	Donna de Lory
3.	MOONLIT HORIZONS	Desert Dwellers
4.	THE WHISPER	Random Lab (ft. Rena)
5.	HIDE AND SEEK	Imogen Heap
6.	WONDERWALL	Ryan Adams
7.	1000 SUNS	Rara Avis
8.	BELOVED (*Thievery Corporation Remix*)	Anoushka Shankar
9.	UDU TU YUTU	Tumbara
10.	SEED	Afro Celt Sound System

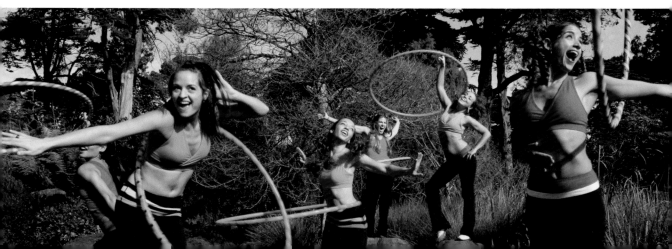

Multiple-Move Fusion

Of the many combinations possible from the moves covered thus far, I've put together a sample routine. Allow yourself to do each move until you feel that the rhythm of the music and the pace of the hoop are complementing one another. Transition (marked with an ▶) from one move to the next only when you feel ready. See pages 189 to 201 for three more routines.

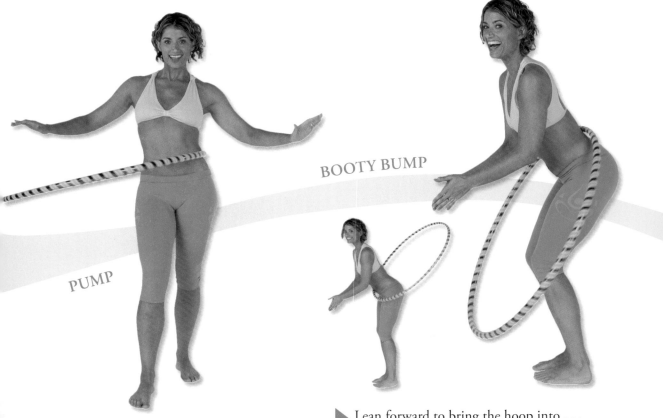

BOOTY BUMP

PUMP

▶ Lean forward to bring the hoop into . . .

1 Start with PUMP. Keep the hoop steady and flat with strong thrusts from your CONTACT POINTS. Lock into the beat of the music and add some simple Step-Touch footsteps (page 27).

2 BOOTY BUMP, popping it up toward the sky with your rear end and bouncing with your heels. Clap your hands as you sync up your BOOTY BUMP with the rhythm.

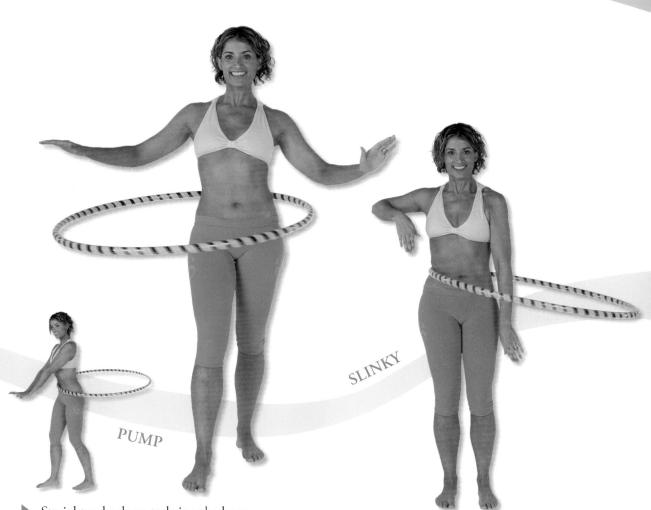

SLINKY

PUMP

▶ Straighten back up to bring the hoop
into . . .

3 PUMP. It may take several rotations
before it resumes a horizontal plane.
Just focus on your posture and your breathing
until it does. Get the PUMP back into rhythm
with the music if it's fallen off.

4 Slow the hoop's rotations slightly by
slowing the pace of your forward-back
push. Focus on the timing of when the hoop
makes contact with you and when the open
spaces between you and the hoop appear. When
you've got the rhythm down, dart your hands in
and out in SLINKY in time with the music.

continued ▶

▶ Multiple-Move Fusion

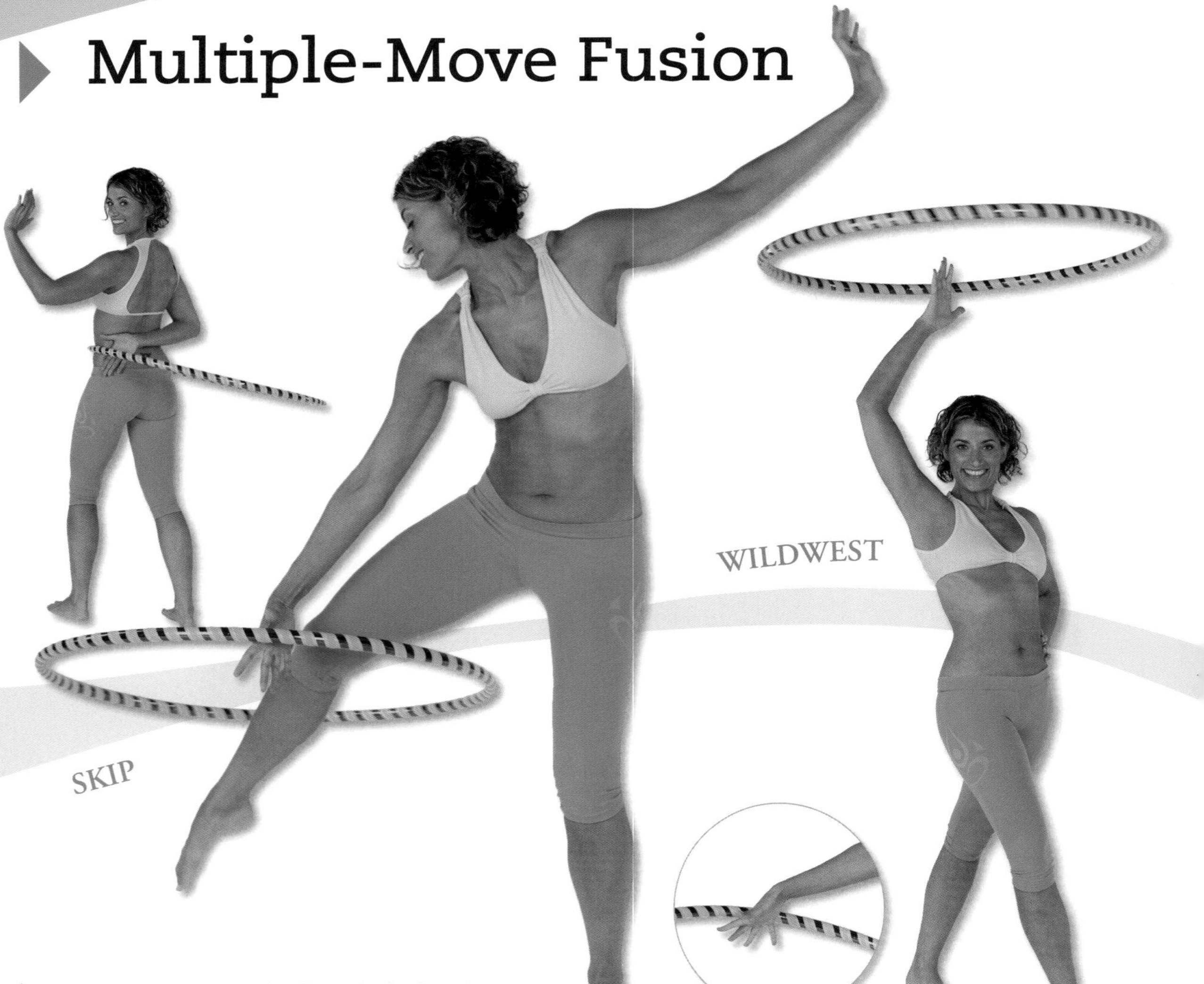

WILDWEST

SKIP

▶ Reach behind your back with the hand opposite from the direction the hoop is moving.

5 Grab the hoop, bring it out in front of you, and tilt it on an angle so you can SKIP out of the hoop. You've elegantly transitioned from your core to off-body. Congratulations!

6 Let the hoop roll over your hand (it's still in the same hand you used for SKIP), and switch your grip so it feels natural. Swing the hoop upward and launch it into WILDWEST above your head. Use assertive push-pull movements to keep the hoop from wobbling.

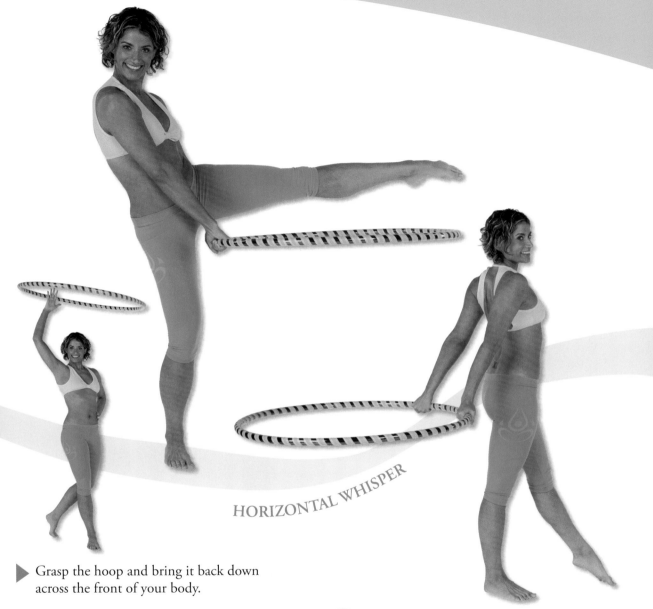

HORIZONTAL WHISPER

▶ Grasp the hoop and bring it back down
across the front of your body.

7   Raise and extend the leg on the
    opposite side of your body and pass
the hoop underneath the raised leg for a
HORIZONTAL WHISPER.

8   Continue to pass the hoop around
    your body on the horizontal plane,
alternating legs as you do more WHISPERS.
It's cool to find a solid beat in your music and
WHISPER each time you hear it.

continued ▶

▶ Multiple-Move Fusion

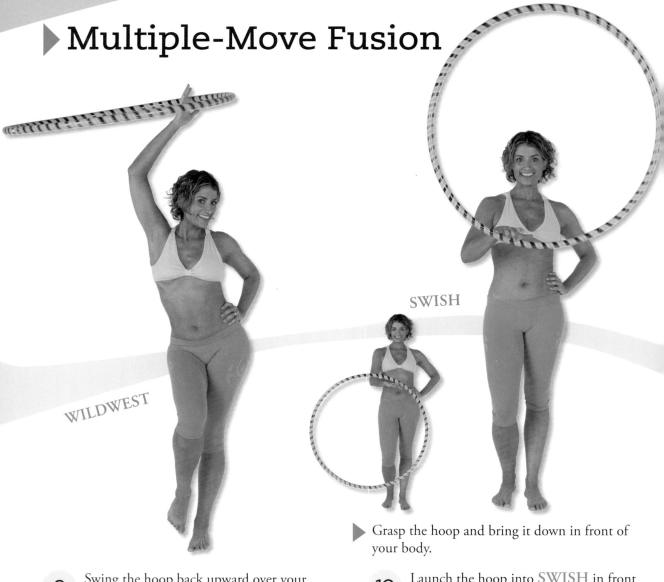

WILDWEST

SWISH

▶ Grasp the hoop and bring it down in front of your body.

9 Swing the hoop back upward over your head and launch into WILDWEST again. Bounce around on your feet, keeping time to the beat.

10 Launch the hoop into SWISH in front of your body. If you're swishing with your right hand, make sure the hoop is moving counterclockwise. If you're using your left hand, the hoop should be moving clockwise.

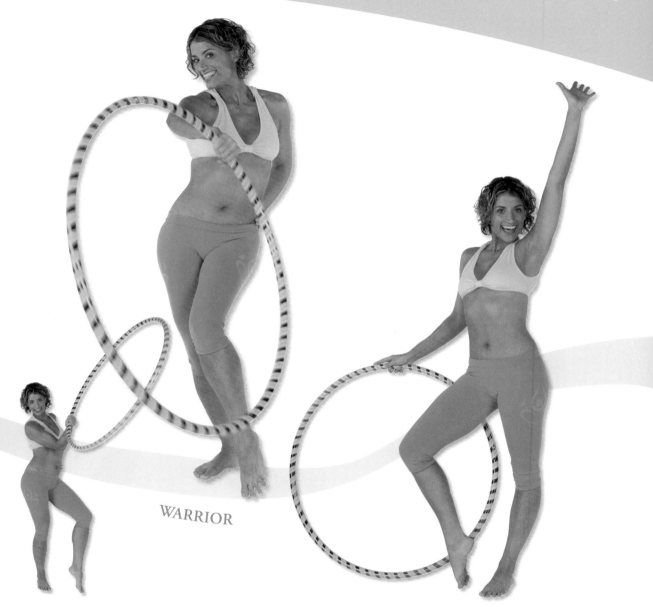

WARRIOR

11 Swing the hoop across your body, into WARRIOR, keeping the hoop vertical and close along the sides of your body. Lean in and out with your shoulders and hips as the hoop moves toward and then away from you.

Finish with flair. Raise the hand not holding the hoop in a triumphant, open-palm *ta-dah!* gesture like an Olympic gymnast, or take a bow! If you're feeling frisky, you can LEAP through the WARRIOR for a smashing finale.

THE PLAYS

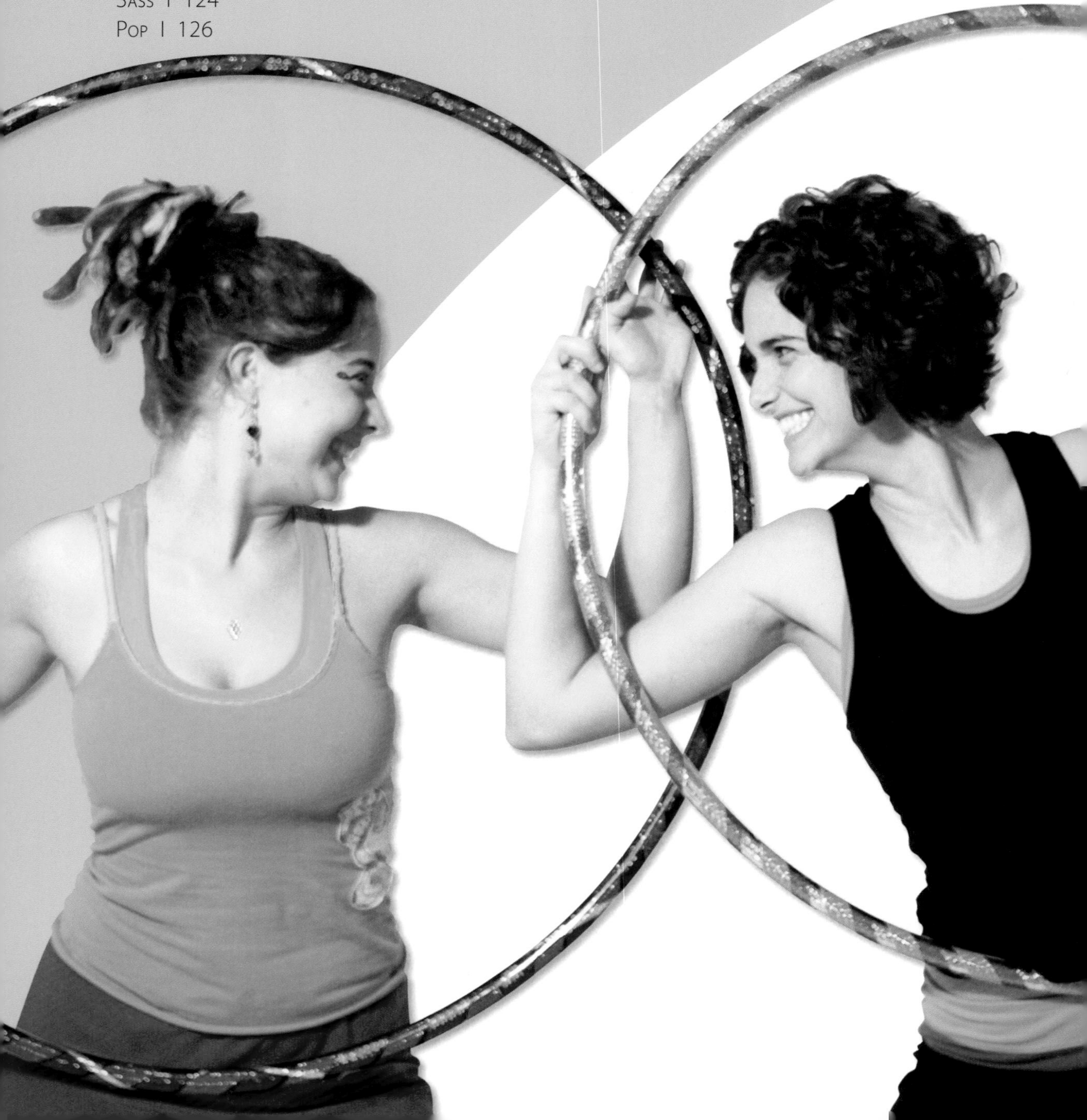

Opposites Attract

CHANGE IT UP WITH
CONTRASTS & REVERSALS

I n the 1950s, the hoop went round and round in one direction. No one was dancing: Just keeping it up was the objective. Today, fancy new tricks are developed by hoop innovators every week and everyone's got their groove on. But these aren't the only differences between then and now. One of the hallmarks of hoopdance today is a joyful exploration of contrast.

That's what this chapter is all about. So get ready for a *challenge*. I like to define a challenge as an invitation to expand my boundaries. Challenges stimulate and exhilarate the mind and heart as much as the body. They make you feel awake, alert, and aware. A move that takes longer to learn teaches you patience and, ultimately, confidence.

Challenging yourself doesn't only mean mastering a new skill; sometimes it's taking a familiar activity and tweaking it. Take a different tack. Explore new sensations. Contrasts in hooping include changing the weight or speed of the hoop, shifting between core hooping and off-body moves, and reversing directions. When you use the muscles on both sides of your body equally, you help prevent injuries.

"As a hip-hop guy, I wanted more back-and-forth rhythm in my hooping to visually reflect the scratching movement of a DJ's turntables. So I brought that rhythm to the hoop by changing its direction, the way a DJ would a record."

—Baxter, 35

Breaking out of cruise control exercises your brain too. Neuroscientist Dr. Larry Katz, coauthor of *Keep Your Brain Alive,* writes that stimulating the brain with unexpected, nonroutine experiences "can actually cause new brain cells to generate . . . and the brain to make new connections between different areas and thus more resistant to the effects of aging." Plus, when your tried-and-true skills suddenly feel fresh

again, you're more likely to stick with your regular hooping practice.

VELOCITY

As you've become more comfortable with Pump, have you noticed your hoop rotating more slowly or faster? There is no right or wrong speed at which to hoop. The right pace is the one that feels good. That said, to challenge yourself, experiment with velocity.

To you speedy types, see how slowly you can go and still keep the hoop in orbit. Speed is often just the *illusion* of mastery: It takes skill to go slowly. Hooping slowly creates space for you to notice nuances. You can consider your fingers, shoulders, toes, and eyes. You can flex each muscle fully. As you relax and slow your breathing, a contemplative calm descends. Your movements might become more sensual. Move in half time with the music, or half as fast as the beat.

If you're on the other end of the spectrum—maybe it's a Bob Marley album that's provided the tempo of *your* hoop sessions—it's time to pick up the pace. Accelerate your forward-back rocking in all the core moves, and swoosh the hoop in off-body moves fast enough to hear wind whistle through the hoop. At this speed, you need to develop agility and precision so you don't lose control of the hoop. Plus you'll blast away calories. To pump you up, find music that seems impossibly fast. Then switch back and forth: slow, then fast, then absolute stillness. Sizzle, simmer, freeze.

TO SEE OR NOT TO SEE

Your eyes transmit a lot of information while you're hooping—such as the position of the hoop in relation to your body, or your posture. A mirror is useful for spotting yourself and improving posture. Your shoulders should be relaxed, pulled back and down. Hold your head high. Notice whether your feet, knees, arms, and hands are in motion. The more of you that is in motion, the better the workout. Also pay attention to the angle of the hoop: In the horizontal moves, it should stay flat without wobbling. Check the angle of your diagonal moves. And while you're at it, check yourself out! Watching yourself glowing while doing PUMP can boost your self-esteem. Or at the very least, it's good for a laugh.

On the flip side, blindfolded hooping magnifies your ability to focus. It teaches you to respond to the feel of the hoop instead of to the sight. You develop a kind of sonar for your posture and balance, so you can *feel* it when you are off center. It's an exhilarating experience to train your body to do a move like the FLOAT UP or WHISPER based entirely on touch. The practice is so good for

developing balance and coordination that it improves your sighted hooping as well.

To try it, grab a bandanna, sleep mask, or a HoopGirl Buff (see page 202). The material should be soft and breathable. Use common sense when choosing a location. Make sure you clear a large space and remove any fragile items. Check for uneven, slippery, or splintery surfaces underfoot, as well as for children or pets. And don't try any moves where you fully release the hoop, like the TOSS!

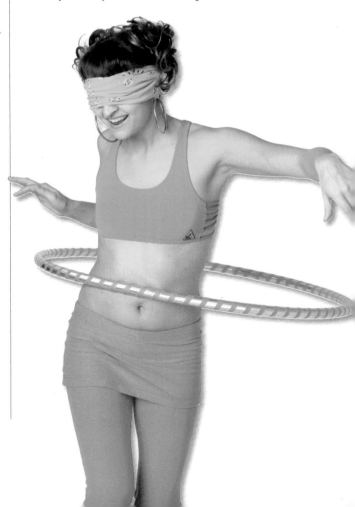

YIN AND YANG

When you meet other hoopers and explore the online hoop community, you might hear the generalization that men hoop faster, with more linear off-body moves, while the feminine style is more flowing and core-based. To relate these contrasts to gender seems limiting, but I do believe you can make hooping more dynamic by exploring yin and yang energy.

Yin energy is slow, soft, gentle, relaxing, surrendering, downward, absorbing, inward, flowing, and liquid. Think of the slow and subtle progress the moon makes through its phases. Move with yielding softness. Rolling, rippling, and swirling are yin movements.

In contrast, yang energy is active, direct, quick, upward and outward, and exciting. Be decisive and bossy as you thrust the hoop through space. Chopping, kicking, leaping, and punching will set yang energy ablaze. Combine both types of energy to keep your muscles and your mind flexible.

GREAT AND SMALL

As you get into more advanced moves, particularly the off-body ones, it may be helpful to use a smaller and lighter hoop. Large hoops rotate more slowly, making it easier to master core moves. A larger, heavier hoop also provides more resistance, which is

HOT AND COLD

You can build your strength as a hooper with hydrotherapy, alternating between hot baths and cold plunges. Switching between hot and cold water rushes your blood around between your core, your extremities, and your skin. It immediately boosts the immune system and soothes muscles. Mineral hot springs are a great place to do this. If you're at home, improvise with a long hot bath with at least two cups of Epsom salts, followed by two minutes of a cold, then hot, then cold shower.

good for pelvic strength and endurance. They lend themselves to smooth, languid, and sensual movement.

Transitioning from a big to a small hoop will return you to that Zen-like "beginner mind," as well as the exhilaration of challenge. Lighter hoops with smaller diameters have more zip. They make off-body moves easier on your arms and hands. Because they're light and rebound more easily, they're better suited to Plays, or reversals in the hoop's direction, which you'll learn in this chapter. See pages 16 and 202 for more information on various sizes of hoops.

Becoming Ambi-hoopstrous

As I mentioned in chapter 2, the direction that your hoop instinctively takes is called your Inflow. Learning to move in the opposite direction, or the Outflow, is the second half of your hooping journey. Going the other way gets you out of your comfort zone and into a whole new world of bidirectional moves. Even though your body has one direction it prefers, it's important to learn to hoop in both directions so you don't develop physical differences on the left and right sides of your body. Mastering your

the glitchy grab bag
PLAYLIST

Trance and Breaks to amplify creativity

1. **BOB N' MARIE** (Mossa Remix) — Joe Ellis
2. **RED ALERT** — Basement Jaxx
3. **SLAP THE BASS** (Original Mix) — Rico Tubbs
4. **ROCKET SOUL** (Original Mix) — Plump DJs
5. **CALYPSO** — Jay Lumen
6. **TOUCH OF MY HAND** (Bill Hamel Club Mix) — Britney Spears
7. **WHAT GOES AROUND . . . COMES AROUND** (Paul van Dyk Club Mix) — Justin Timberlake
8. **SMALL STEP ON THE OTHER SIDE** (Elevation Remix) — Basic Pespective
9. **TERRA TRONICS** — Protoculture
10. **RIDE** (Tiesto Extended Remix) — Cary Brothers

Outflow also happens to be a building block for Play, the intermediate concept we cover in this chapter. So practice up. It's playtime!

Play

To Play the hoop is to stop the flow of its rotation and send it moving in the opposite direction. Playing is a concept rather than a move, because it can be applied to most moves. It can also be done using a variety of body parts such as elbows and knees, as well as from inside the hoop, although here we'll simply be using a hand on the outside of the hoop.

PLAY YOUR PUMP

While in Pump catch the hoop with one hand and push it in the opposite direction. The challenge is to keep the hoop on its original plane without wobbling once you've reversed its direction.

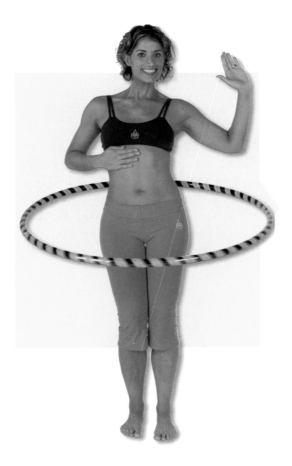

1 Start in Pump. Focus on the rhythm of the hoop. You will be stopping its rotation just before it disappears behind you, at the edge of your peripheral vision, using the hand on that side of your body. So if the hoop is moving to your left, Play it on the left side of your body, using your left hand.

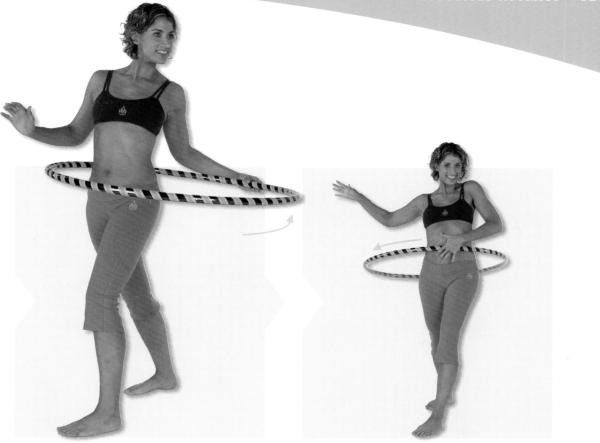

2 Catch the hoop on the *outside*. Keep the hand and arm supple and receptive, twisting your torso to go *with* the hoop (like when you catch a ball) as it continues moving in its original direction a few more degrees.

3 Then push the hoop into your core so it swings back into PUMP, heading in the opposite direction. Now PUMP the hoop in your OUTFLOW. If your original direction was to your left, the hoop should now be rotating toward your right.

a tip for triumph

▶ To keep each PLAY from being wobbly, really twist your spine to follow the hoop as it slows in your grasp. Then give it an assertive push to send it back into a strong horizontal orbit.

Garter, Bun & Boing!

Here's a way to PLAY the hoop during SWISH. Use the surface of the thigh (GARTER), butt (BUN), or foot (BOING!) to reverse the direction of the hoop.

NOTE: Use the thigh/bun/foot on the same side of your body as the hoop is rotating.

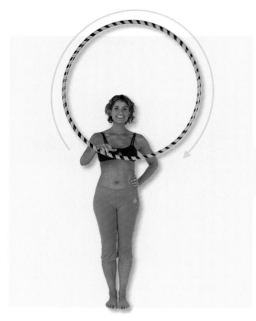

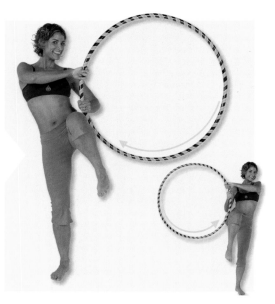

Start in SWISH (page 66)**.** As the hoop rotates downward, use the strength in your hand— at the instant you grasp the hoop in your palm—to begin slowing its rotation.

For GARTER: As the hoop approaches your thigh, lift your knee up to make a 90 degree angle so that your thigh provides a surface for the hoop to bounce off. Bring the other hand on the hoop to assist and let the hoop bounce off the outer part of your thigh. Presto! You are now SWISHING in the opposite direction.

variations

▶ You can also use the *inner* thigh to do GARTER. To do so, lift the knee on the side of your body *opposite* the direction the hoop is rotating. Similarly, you can use the *inner* side of your foot for BOING!

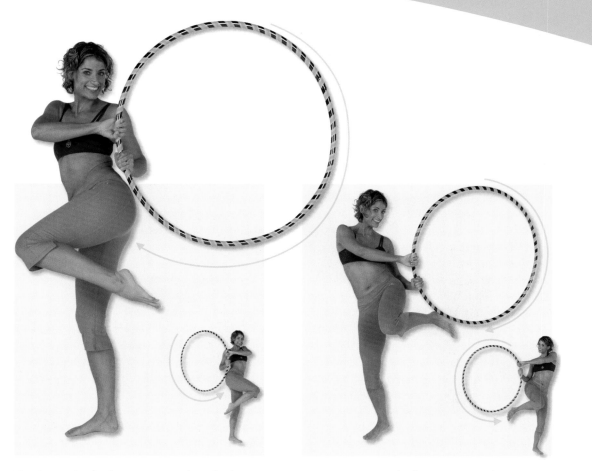

For Bun: As the hoop approaches the hip, twist your pelvis so the side of your hip/bun faces forward (keep your upper body facing straight ahead). Allow the hoop to bounce off your butt and ricochet back in the opposite direction. The direction of your Swish should now be reversed.

For Boing!: As the hoop approaches your foot, lift your knee and angle it slightly inward (toward the opposite knee) to expose the outer side of the foot. Slowing the rotation with your hand(s), lightly tap the hoop on the outside of your foot. (The hoop should have slowed enough that it hardly impacts your foot.)

Sass

An off-body move in which the hoop is held horizontally and Played off the hips to reverse its direction.

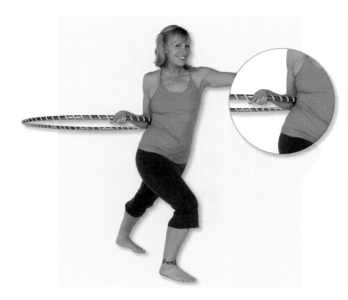
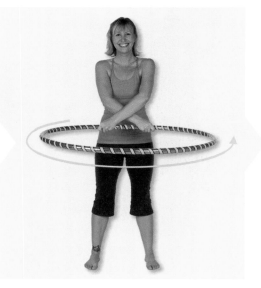

1 Hold the hoop on your right side on the horizontal plane. Grip it on the inside and let it rest on your right hip, using your forearm and elbow to secure it, as shown.

2 Swing the hoop toward your left. As it moves in front of you, grasp the hoop with your left hand so your wrists cross (left on top) and for a moment both hands are on the hoop, pinky facing pinky.

DANCE-IFY IT

Explore space with your free hand and look over your shoulder as you twist. Add dynamism by stepping back with the foot opposite the hoop.

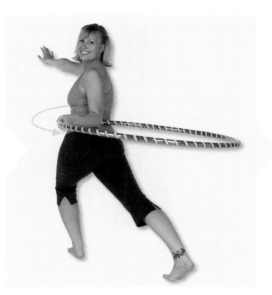

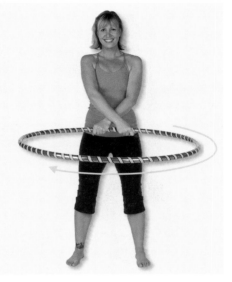

3 Release your right hand, and allow the momentum of the hoop to continue its swing to your left. Twist your torso to the left to allow the hoop to travel farther. When the hoop makes contact with the back of your hip, allow that impact to send it in the opposite direction—to your right.

4 As the hoop passes in front of you going in the opposite direction, reach your right hand in and grasp the hoop so your wrists are crossed again, this time with your right on top.

5 Release the left hand and allow the hoop to swing to your right, twisting your torso, until the hoop PLAYS off your right hip and back. Continue PLAYING from side to side.

Pop

An intermediate off-body move in which the hoop is held horizontally and bounced off the upper arms to reverse its direction.

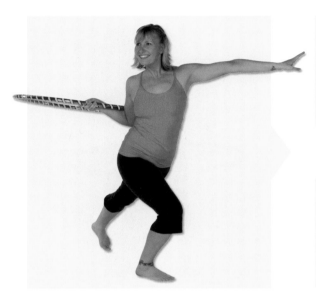

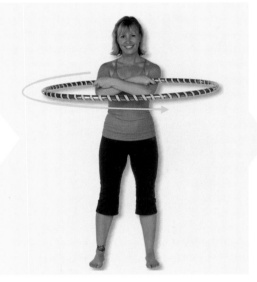

1 Begin with the hoop held off the body in the horizontal plane, on your right side, with your right hand. Keep your arm bent, so that the hoop rests on your forearm and is tucked into your inner elbow. (You need a lot of wrist strength to hold this position.)

2 Keeping the hoop flat (horizontal), swing it to your left side. As it passes in front of you, reach your left hand under and inside the hoop so that your forearms cross.

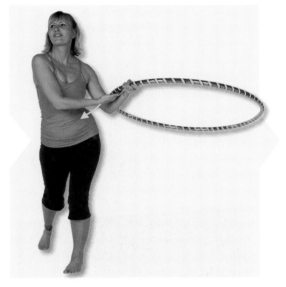

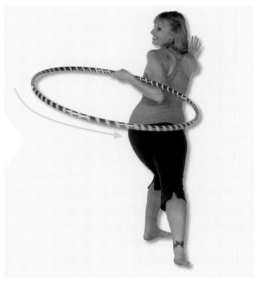

3 Quickly release the right hand, pulling it out from being crossed with the left. The hoop is now in your left hand, in a grip that is the mirror image of the starting position of step 1.

4 Allow the left hand and forearm to continue swinging the hoop to the left side of your body. Twist your torso to allow the hoop to travel as far as possible to your left.

5 When the hoop makes contact with your left triceps, allow it to bounce off and reverse direction. The hoop now is moving back toward the right side of your body (in your left hand).

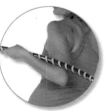

Repeat steps 1–5 in reverse, with the hoop PLAYING off your right triceps.

A Study in Contrasts

YES, I'M A GUY. THERE ARE QUITE A FEW male hoopers actually. I "grew up hooping," as I like to say, a few years back in San Luis Obispo, where most of the hoopers were men. And I'm talking manly men. One of them, my friend Grant, is a burly construction worker.

I'm an architect by trade and by passion. So I'm not a kinesthetic learner—I understand things spatially. What excites me about hooping is creating shapes in space. I actually make diagrams of things I dream up to do with a hoop, and then I try to realize them. I've had some ideas that I haven't been physically able to do yet.

I had this *aha!* moment after watching a video of myself hooping. In the video I hooped really fast the whole time. The funny thing was, when you watched it, you couldn't really tell it was so fast because there was nothing to compare it to. So now I play a lot with changing speeds, reversing directions, and isolating the hoop in one spot. For me, isolation is the lack of contrast; it's like when a camera lens pauses to find its focus. It is the space between the words. The pauses are critical emphases that help construct the rhythm.

It amazes me how hooping has evolved: In the 1950s there were hardly any contrasting elements. The hoop just went around and around in one direction. Today lots of hoopers make their directional changes into beats, rhythms, and tempos. This is what keeps it interesting.

I also like to play little visual jokes. A joke is when a person has an expectation, and then the joker does something completely unexpected. When hooping, I establish a rhythm and cadence. But then I can break out of it, as a sudden surprise. That's another contrast: the difference between the expected and what actually happens with my hoop.

What can I say? I'm a complete geek when it comes to hooping.

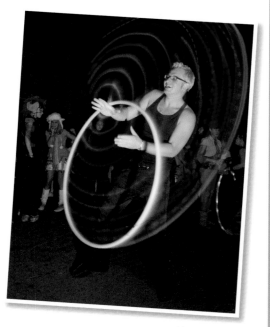

Name: Rich
Occupation: Architect

"If I had to hoop for long in just one direction, I would feel completely unbalanced. This has to do with balancing my two halves: my right brain and my left brain, my feminine self and my masculine self, my dark side and my light side. I love the call-and-answer feeling of changing directions. It is a percussive conversation that juxtaposes, blurs, and softens the dissonances I want to resolve within myself."

—Beth, 43

Wheel of Life Journal Exercise

Draw a circle in your journal. Divide it into six wedges like a pie. Label each of the six sections with the following words: 1) Work, 2) Exercise, 3) Friends, 4) Romance, 5) Play, 6) Spirituality. Inside each segment, make a dot. If you are very fulfilled and rich in that area, put the dot near the outside of the circle. If you're not very fulfilled in that area, put it near the center. Now connect the dots.

What kind of a shape is formed by the connected dots? If it looks like a circle, it means your life is balanced. If so, how big is your circle? Can it get any bigger? If the shape looks more like a mutant star, maybe there are areas of your life that need enriching. What kinds of activities could you do to move the innermost dots toward the outer ring?

Circles have been used since ancient times to represent unity and wholeness. It's fitting to use this one to see how complete your life is, and where the holes are! And of course standing in the center of one—your hoop—and keeping it balanced in orbit also ties into the rich symbolism of the circle. You never know: Over time, the hoop might help you gain more balance between the various elements in your life.

THE MOVES

The Pursuit of Hoopiness

PLAYFUL SPINSATIONS

Hooping is like a miracle cure-all. Pretty much everyone who gets the hoop going in Pump describes a positive emotional rush, using words like *exhilaration, bliss, triumph,* and *joy*. Then there are the hoop's glorious effects on your muscle tone, making you feel stronger and leaner. There's the comforting feeling of the hoop continuously massaging your core, which trains your body to seek out the feel-good sensation and sustain it for longer and longer periods of time. There may be an awakening of the sensual and flirtatious parts of you. And then there's the serene, meditative aspect of Pump that quiets the mind—making you feel centered and grounded.

Really, it's simple: Hooping makes you happy. The playfulness of gyration is inherently joyful. This is useful information, since studies show that more than one out of every five women in the U.S. will become clinically depressed during her lifetime. Psychologist and author Dr. Richard Holden says that "a happy person is not a person in a certain set of circumstances, but rather a person with a certain set of attitudes." Happy people accept themselves as good enough, see setbacks as temporary, and stay optimistic in difficult situations. So when the hoop teaches you to say, "Yes, I can!" *(I can keep it up! I can recover it when it starts to fall! With some effort I know I can master this move!),* it's a mind-set you can apply in all areas of life. Yes, you can.

For me, hooping reminds me that life is good. The hoop pressing on my body pushes a wake-up button within me. Even when my hooping is fierce, fast, and strong, it still softens something inside me. It helps me let go. When I step out of the hoop, my

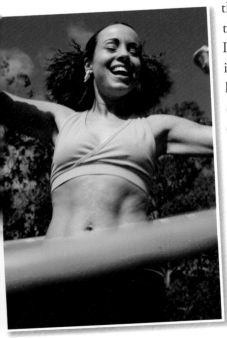

thoughts linger on the joy I feel and I try to sustain it in my everyday life—washing the dishes, working, even walking down the street.

Hoopers have told me that they are literally unable to stay in a bad mood while

fantastic tunes
PLAYLIST

Theatrical and silly tunes to transport you to new worlds.

1.	**AMADO MIO**	Pink Martini
2.	**SEXY BITCHES**	Amae
3.	**I CAN'T DO IT ALONE**	*Chicago* (film sound track)
4.	**BABY FACE**	Marissa Jaret Winokur
5.	**TRUE LOVE'S KISS**	*Enchanted* (film sound track)
6.	**HONEY ROCK**	Barney Kessel & Gloria Wood
7.	**WHEN YOU'RE GOOD TO MAMA**	*Chicago* (film sound track)
8.	**I WANNA BE LOVED BY YOU**	Helen Kane
9.	**RIGHT NOW**	The Pussycat Dolls
10.	**CANDYMAN**	Christina Aguilera

spinning inside their hoop. The movement expels nervous energy and calms the insecurities that can lead to fear, jealousy, or bitterness. As Abby, a publicist in Florida, says, "Hooping is the best therapy! On bad days I hoop, and then my mood changes for the better. I'm able to just be in the moment, with the reassuring push-pull of the hoop

What If . . .

Using any and all of the moves you've mastered, let's play pretend! Imagine you're Supergirl, blasting off into the air to right wrongs. Use your hoop as a cape! Or become a Carneval dancer in Rio, crowned in a headdress of fabulous feathers, doing BOOTY BLITZ with persuasive percussion. Or you're an Amazonian warrior priestess in a bronze-fronted bodice, raising your hoop to the sky like a staff before launching it into WARRIOR. Imagine you're a gossamer-winged fairy, sprinkling glitter with your hoop as it circles you in NECTAR.

Now imagine that your body is composed of different elements other than flesh and blood. What if you were made of falling leaves, blooming flowers, flames, water, or pure sunshine? What if you were a cloud, a piece of seaweed, a feather carried by a breeze, an ocean wave? How do these images inspire you to use your arms differently? Your head? Your fingers? Let these images animate your whole body.

cradling me. I lose all sense of time and just meditate within the blissful vortex."

All Fun and Games

You can't deny that hooping reminds you of being a kid again. In this chapter I invite you into the deep end of the kiddie pool to play, and into the realms of fantasy and make-believe. The bell for recess is ringing, so use the hoop as your transporter and pop through the rabbit hole. I mean, hooping's already pretty wacky, so it's not such a stretch to take it a few steps further, right?

The moves in this chapter are specially engineered for adventure and fun. It takes confidence to goof around and be silly. You have to take a risk and become vulnerable. You have to forget about what other people might think. Letting go of control is actually a radical statement of courage.

So hold onto your (imaginary) hat! These moves are as whimsical as they are athletic. Some have kooky sound effects. You'll use your feet like hands and your shoulders like shelves and your elbows like paintbrushes. Come on now, I double dare you!

Revolving Door

During this move, the hoop is held vertically off the body and swung around your body for you to step through. REVOLVING DOOR always makes me think of leprechauns, hobbits, and gnomes—magical creatures that pop up unexpectedly!

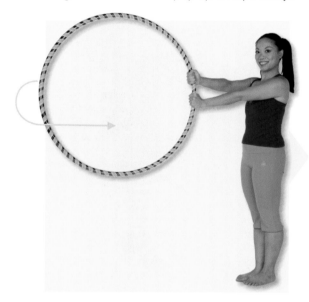

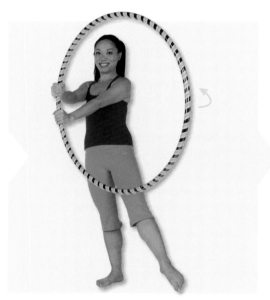

1 Start by holding the hoop vertically in front of you with both hands close together—pinky of one facing the thumb of the other. Keep a loose grip in one place on the hoop so that it can swivel in a full circle. Your hands are the axis on which you turn the hoop.

2 Keeping your arms stationary, swivel the hoop so the edge opposite your grip swings around your body.

---

a tip for triumph

▶ Keep the hoop relatively high, a few feet off the ground. To pass the first leg through the REVOLVING DOOR at this height, exhale deeply and engage your abdominals. Extend each leg fully, pointing your toes.

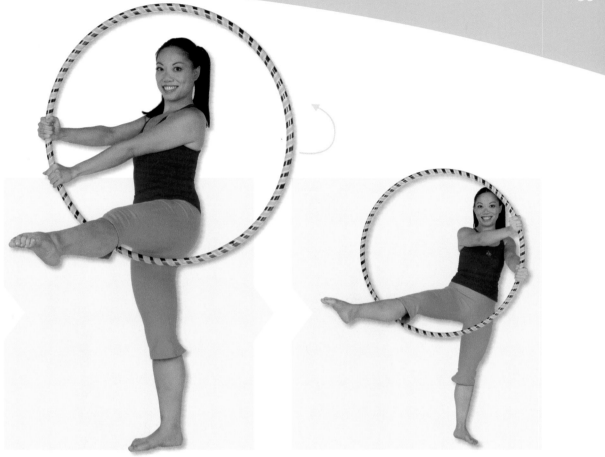

3 If the hoop is moving to your left, lift and pass your left leg through the hoop, then duck your head and step through quickly with the other foot. (Do the opposite if the hoop is moving to your right.) Imagine passing through a magical doorway, like Alice into Wonderland.

4 Maintaining your loose grip, continue to swivel the hoop so it circles around your body. You can pass through the REVOLVING DOOR again and again, or change directions.

Whoopee!

Jump up and pass the vertical hoop between your legs from the hand in front to the hand behind you.

NOTE: Before doing this move, measure your vertical hoop against your pants' inseam to be sure that the hoop can pass between your legs. If not, use a smaller hoop.

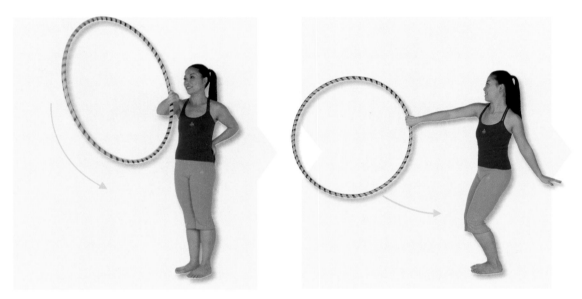

1 The hoop's starting position for WHOOPEE! is similar to REVOLVING DOOR'S, but you're going to need some momentum. So get the hoop going in WARRIOR.

2 While swinging the hoop forward across your body, bring it toward your centerline rather than crossing it in front of you to your opposite side.

vocalize

▶ Try shouting out "whooooppeee!" as you do this move. Notice how your voice can intensify the energy in your jump and make you go higher.

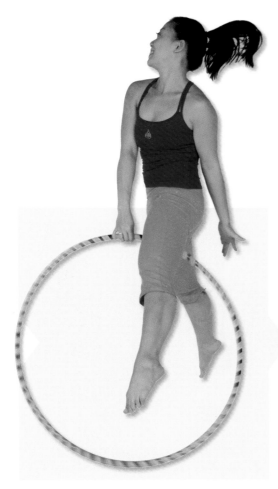

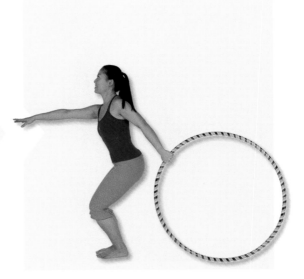

3 Engage your abs and bend your knees to spring-load your legs, then jump directly upward with both feet, as high as you can, while simultaneously swinging the hoop between your legs. Just like in a jumping jack, scissor your legs out to the sides as you get airborne.

4 When the hoop is directly underneath you and between your legs, grab it near your butt with the opposite hand. (Your hands should face thumb to thumb.) Release the hoop so it ends up behind you in the second hand, still on the vertical plane.

Bling

Starting with the hoop in front of you, bring it backward over your head to pop it off your rear, then forward to bounce off your thighs.

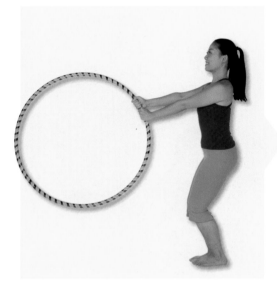 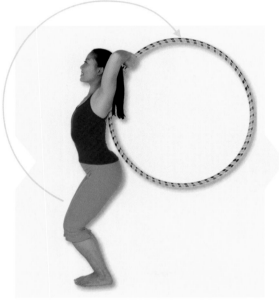

1 Using both hands, hold the hoop on the vertical directly in front of you. Your hands should be next to each other, pinky to thumb. Stand with your feet together and your knees slightly bent.

2 Bring the hoop up and backward, directly over your head. Stick your butt out to provide a surface for the hoop to bounce off.

DANCE-IFY IT

Create a beautiful S shape in your body by bending your knees and arching your back as the hoop makes contact with your butt.

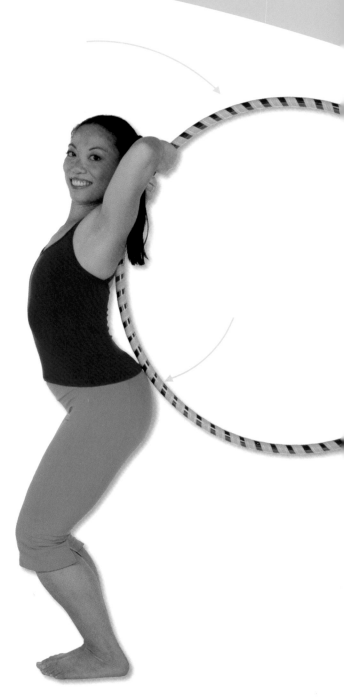

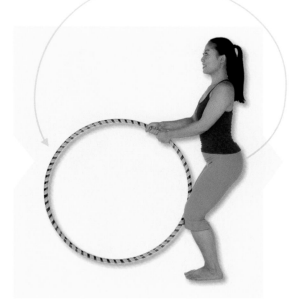

3 After it bounces, bring the hoop back down to where it started. As the hoop descends, bend a little deeper at the knees, press your thighs tightly together, and allow the hoop to bounce off their surface, then back up and over your head.

Carousel

Use your foot to carry the hoop partway around your body on the horizontal plane.

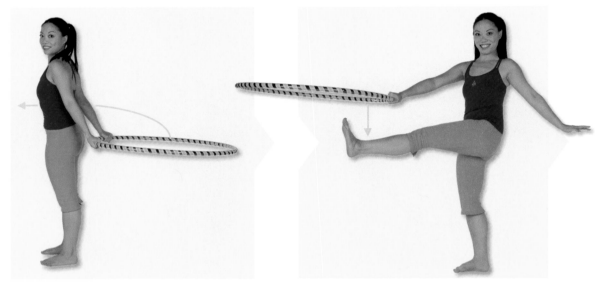

1 Start in NECTAR (page 68). As you bring the hoop around to the front, engage your abs and leg muscles to lift and extend one leg (the one opposite your hoop arm) in front of you.

2 Create an L shape by flexing the foot of the lifted leg and pulling your toes toward your shin. This creates a hook for carrying the hoop.

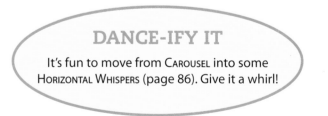

DANCE-IFY IT

It's fun to move from CAROUSEL into some HORIZONTAL WHISPERS (page 86). Give it a whirl!

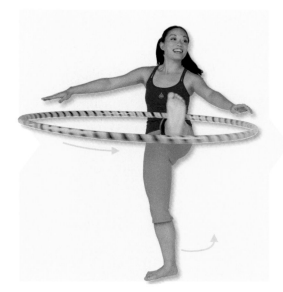

3 Place the hoop over your foot so it's held by the hook of your ankle, and immediately move that leg in the direction the hoop has been moving. Swing the leg quickly to keep the hoop from drooping. Hop in the same direction with the standing foot.

4 Bring the leg as far around the side of the body as you can and still have it feel good.

5 When your foot can't carry the hoop any further, grasp the hoop with your hand, palm-down and carry it around the back of your body so it completes a full circle.

Bingo

Bingo is like Carousel, except you use your knee to hook and carry the hoop horizontally as you twirl.

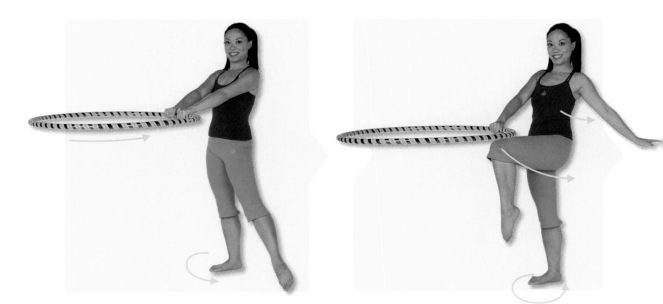

1 Start in Nectar (page 68). Take steps to turn your body in the direction the hoop is moving to build momentum.

2 Lift the knee opposite the hand holding the hoop. Engage your abs to protect your lower back. Lift the knee as high as possible to act as a hook for the hoop. Keep turning.

be aware!

▶ Bingo can make you dizzy. Start slow with short spins and breathe deeply. Another way to reduce dizziness is to "spot" an object in the room by returning your gaze to that same place every time you turn.

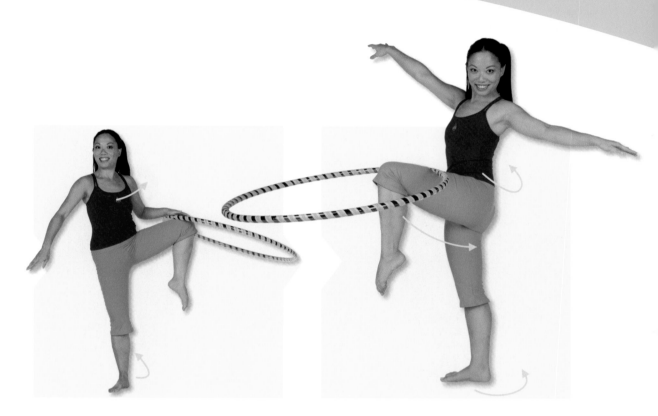

3 Place the hoop on the hook of your knee so it's resting on your thigh. Get used to the sensation by holding the hoop in place on your thigh while you spin.

Pivot and then hop on the standing foot to spin as long as you can while carrying the hoop on the raised leg.

4 Release your hand! You need to spin *fast* to keep the hoop from drooping. Aim to keep the hoop as close to horizontal as possible while it's suspended. When you can't spin any further, remove the hoop with your hand and lower your knee.

• The more you practice, the more you'll develop counterbalancing skills as you whirl.

Jingle

In JINGLE the hoop rotates around your bent elbow on the surface of your upper arm and forearm.

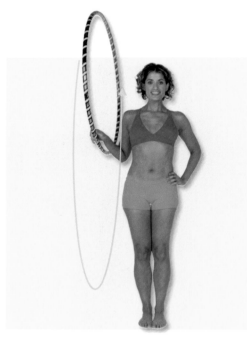

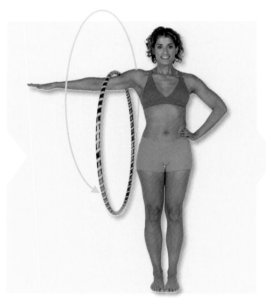

1 Start in SWISH (page 66) and turn so you're SWISHING along the side of your body rather than in front of you. Allow the hoop to get some momentum.

2 Stick your SWISHING arm inside until the hoop is revolving around your biceps and triceps. Keep the hoop rotating by making circles with your whole arm from the shoulder, pushing into the hoop as you feel it press against you.

visualize
▶ Imagine there's a paintbrush attached to your elbow and you're painting an egg shape with it.

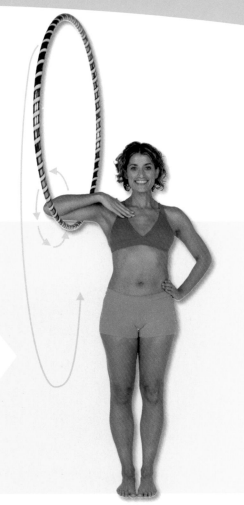

3 When you can, bend your arm at the elbow, bringing your hand to your shoulder. (Your elbow should be pointing out to the side, with the tip slightly raised.) Experiment to find just the right angle.

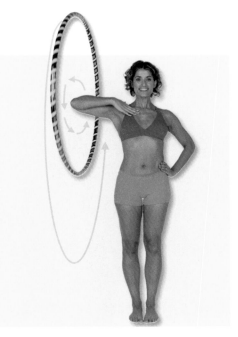

4 Keep rotating the hoop by making circles with your bent arm, pushing against the hoop when you feel it pressing into you. To remove the hoop, simply open your hand and grasp the hoop on the inside and continue SWISHING.

• Practice JINGLE on both elbows, with the hoop rotating both to the right and to the left on each.

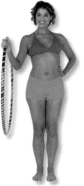

Fling

Toss the hoop up into the air, using your elbow.

NOTE: Make sure you are outdoors or in a space with at least fourteen-foot ceilings.

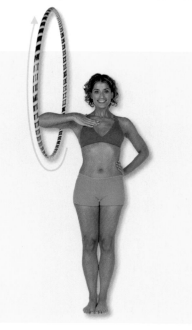

1 Start in JINGLE with the hoop swinging forward and up. Watch the hoop's rotation around your elbow to see when it starts its upward rotation. Notice the sensations on your arm when the hoop is on the upswing versus coming back down.

2 When you next feel the hoop on the top of your arm, create a U-shaped movement with your elbow by dipping it down and then straight upward in one assertive motion. Add some oomph to the toss by bending your knees.

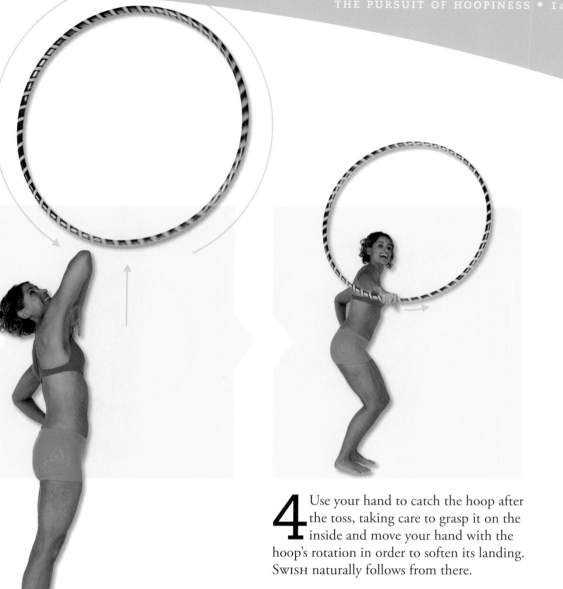

4 Use your hand to catch the hoop after the toss, taking care to grasp it on the inside and move your hand with the hoop's rotation in order to soften its landing. SWISH naturally follows from there.

3 Toss the hoop off your elbow straight up in the air. Pop up with your whole body at the moment of the launch.

Sparkle

Flip the hoop on a circular path under the armpit so it flies over the shoulder from back to front, and then down the front of the body.

NOTE: Instructions are for right-handers. Reverse them if you're a lefty.

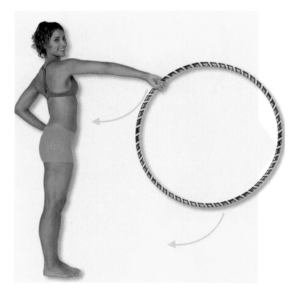

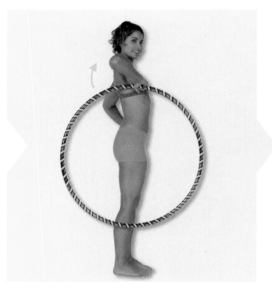

1 Begin in WARRIOR (page 72) using your right hand. As the hoop swings back to your right side, turn your wrist slightly so the hoop can swing straight back under your right arm on the vertical.

2 Swing the hoop under your right armpit, extending your hand as far back as it can go before releasing.

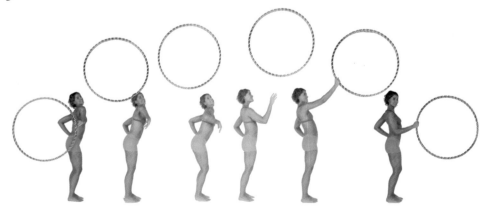

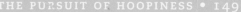

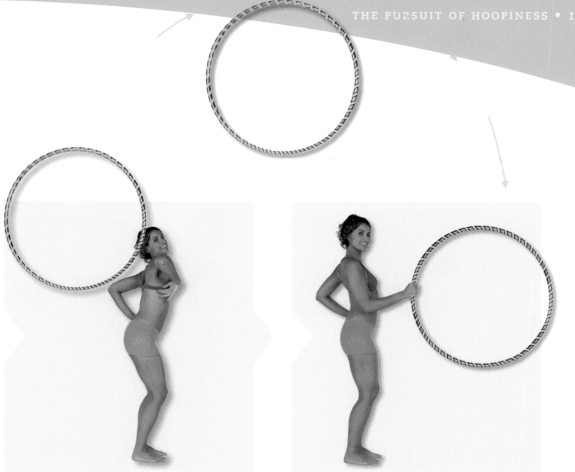

3 When you release the hoop, use your fingers to give it an extra push and send it into a spin. The hoop should spin up behind and over the top of your right shoulder, so it flies in front of you. It may help to lean forward at the moment you release so that gravity helps pull the hoop to your front.

4 Extend your hand and grab the hoop on its descent. Grab it on the inside, with your thumb pointing up.

DANCE-IFY IT

After a SPARKLE, the hoop will flow smoothly back into SWISH (page 66) alongside your body. Let your feet patter in rhythm with the music.

Libra

Rest the hoop atop one shoulder and turn continuously, allowing the momentum of your body to "carry" the hoop on a near-horizontal plane.

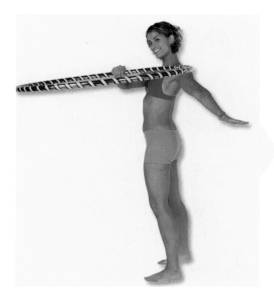

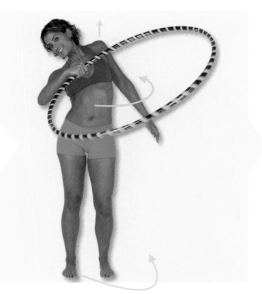

1 Pick a shoulder—the one that you can lift higher. Start with the hoop horizontal, held in the hand opposite your chosen shoulder. Move the hoop up toward the shoulder as though you're about to do PEARL (page 70).

2 Lift the shoulder up, leaning the opposite shoulder toward the ground to make the surface atop your shoulder into as much of a "shelf" for the hoop as possible.

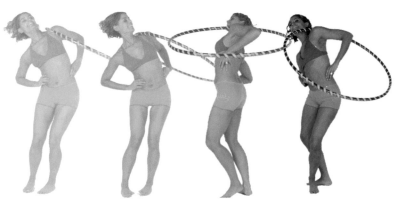

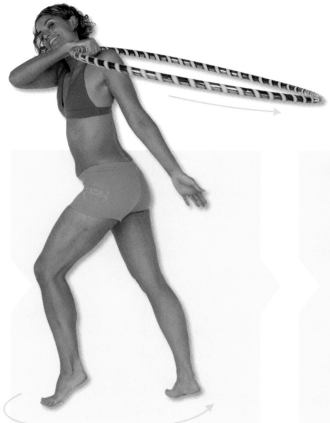

3 Lay the hoop on your shoulder and release the hand that placed it there. Keep your shoulder high. Immediately start turning your body by taking small, quick steps.

4 The faster you spin, the more horizontal the hoop will become. Imagine you have a precious gem perched atop your shoulder—keep it from slipping off at all costs!

variation
▶ If you can't get the hoop to stay on its "shelf," place your hand on the side of your head. This creates a loop that holds the hoop in place.

Getting in the Hoop Loop

If your world is crowded with friends, I bet you've told them about hooping. Maybe you've persuaded some of them to try it; maybe you've gotten one to buy a hoop; maybe you've even been giving lessons. If you haven't, think about it! Hoops have universal appeal. They make great icebreakers at parties. Sometimes it's the people you least expect to give it a whirl or swing their hips who just can't put the hoop down—probably the ones who most need some silliness and gyration in their lives.

If you're looking to expand your circles, hooping opens lots of avenues. There may already be a hoop group in your area that brings locals together to jam, swap moves and tricks, and share their passion for the hoop. Every hoop group I've ever encountered has been friendly and noncompetitive, welcoming folks off the street who want to try a hoop for the first time ever. They usually represent all skill levels, all body types, and all walks of life. Hooping.org, the world's international online hooping hub, lists all active groups with their contact information. Visit it to connect up with other hoopers in your neighborhood and to get the scoop on news in the hoop universe.

If there isn't a hoop group near you, consider starting one! The easiest way is to head out to a park or open public space with some extra hoops and music—and any other hoopers you've already met. People passing by will be magnetized and soon you'll be surrounded by new hooping friends. Get their e-mail addresses so you can let them know about the next meet-up. Presto: a new hoop group!

Now that you're in the loop, you'll suddenly notice people carrying cheerful neon hoops around the way people carry yoga mats. Events such as music festivals and outdoor theater or concerts are great places to bring your hoop and meet other hoopers. Every year that passes there are more and more hooping-specific gatherings—retreats and workshops like the Hoop Path and Hoop Convergence in North Carolina or the Hoop Camp in California. These events give you the opportunity to study with the biggest names in hooping, like Hoopaliscious, Spiral, Baxter, and Bunny Hoop Star (who hails from Australia!).

Who knows whether hooping would have become the international phenomenon

performance as
TRANSFORMANCE

There's absolutely no need and no rush for you to take the stage with your hoop, but I do want to share some of the revelations I've had while performing. In 2005, when I made weekly appearances under the sparkling lights of the biggest nightclub in San Francisco, I'd look out from the stage to the screaming hordes reaching out to me. While connecting to the primal thumping beat and interacting with the audience, I discovered parts of myself I didn't know were in me. I had to overcome fear, be willing to be seen, and accept adoration and praise.

I suddenly understood that performance was about transmitting emotions to the audience, and I began focusing on generating specific energies—projecting joy, love, hope, faith. My biggest realization was that the qualities you need to appear on stage—courage, poise, knowing how to "fake it 'til you make it" and how to truly connect with people around you—are the same skills you need to "appear" and succeed in any setting.

If you can play, you can perform! Perform in front of a mirror! Perform in a jam circle with a bunch of hooping friends! It doesn't matter how many tricks you know—it's all about sharing your enthusiasm and joy. If you reveal your radiance to others, you will always receive appreciation.

So take the feel-good factor that hooping automatically brings you and let it out, let it show, let it shine. Use your posture and your breath to convey qualities such as strength and courage, innocence and wonder, or spiritual groundedness and connection. Use your eyes and mouth to communicate things like surprise, jubilation, flirtation, or longing. Tell whatever story feels authentic to you—performing is just another way of telling your story.

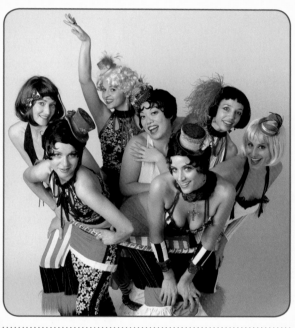

The HoopGirl Allstars

Neuroscience by Day, Hooping by Night

BY DAY, I'M A METHODICAL, DETAIL-ORIENTED research assistant in the neuroscience department at the University of California at Berkeley. My lab studies memory using behavioral tests and brain scans. It's fascinating and challenging, but it involves a lot of time sitting in front of a computer.

Hooping, on the other hand, gives my body its challenge. Just getting out of my chair and giving the hoop a spin in my office shakes the numbness from my limbs and puts me in touch with my body. After I had made hooping my serious (yet silly) passion for over a year, Christabel invited me to join her performance troupe,

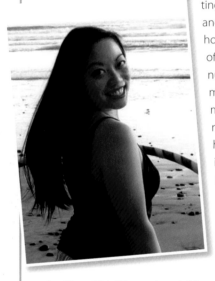

the HoopGirl Allstars. In addition to my own personal practice hours, I rehearse with the troupe for two hours every week and perform almost weekly at parties and nightclubs.

As a thirty-something woman with a demanding day job, I no longer stay out at bars until the wee hours. My work wardrobe is functional and understated: jeans nearly every day. So hoopdancing is an excuse to transform myself—to break out the glitter, mile-long eyelashes, and fantastical outfits. It lets me explore my playful side, and not just by donning a costume. I can become a glamorous goddess with long faux tresses and some languid, gracious arm gestures. With a tilt of my head, a bobbed wig, and my feet kicking up a Charleston step, I transform into a flirty flapper. Or I can zip around and wave my hoop to scatter magic glitter like Tinker Bell.

For a nerd like me, hooping is a way to stretch my imagination and my body at the same time.

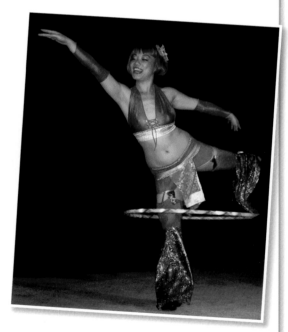

Name: Natasha
Occupation: Neuroscience Researcher

it is without the help of the Internet. Many hoopers are on social networks such as Facebook and tribe.net and have created special groups around hoop-linked topics, from outfits and tricks to spiritual breakthroughs and music. YouTube and other popular sites host literally thousands of hooping videos. Hoopers use these online videos to learn new moves and inspire new combinations. I'm always amazed to find a new video by a woman in Finland or Alaska who learned everything she knows on the Internet.

All in all, I'd be surprised if hooping doesn't broaden your social circles . . . if you want it to. Playing with others really amplifies the giddiness, sassiness, and fun factor of your hooping. The hours just fly by while hooping with friends.

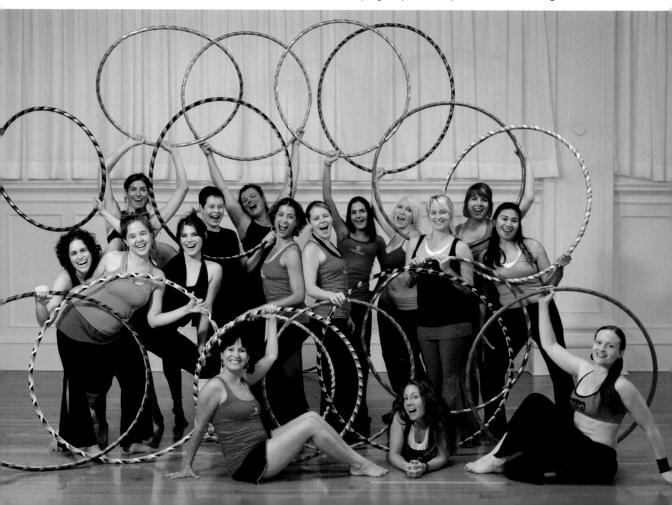

Hooping it up at a HoopGirl Teacher Training

THE MOVES

The Smoothest Moves

INVITE YOUR INNER SEX GODDESS OUT TO PLAY

The hoop is a dance partner like no other—one that wraps itself around you with the same tenacious glee whether you're PMS-ing in saggy gray sweatpants or at the top of your game in an itty-bitty bikini. It's a trusty partner that never steps on your feet and always comes back around, one that responds to your every move—even the tiniest shift in posture—and keeps perfect time. So even if you've always felt like a klutz on the dance floor or have no natural rhythm, hooping will help you get your groove on.

Responsiveness, repetition, and rhythm . . . what else comes to mind? Hooping makes you feel *sexy*! It rocks your hips and gets the blood moving in your pelvis. It taps into a primal energy within you, a raw vitality. In the hoop you become unabashedly fluid, sensual, and wild. When you're in that place, you glow.

But in our culture, the word *sexy* has been stolen by the people who peddle it— the fashion, cosmetic, and pharmaceutical companies who make it about how you look rather than how you *feel*. One of my goals both in my classes and in this book is to redefine *sexy*. It's not about 32-24-35. Sexy is about grace and presence, about exuding self-love, poise, and confidence. Sexy is an energetic radiance that anyone of any age, gender, or body shape can tap into. You just have to discover these qualities within yourself and *own* them. And that's what hooping helps you do.

The sexiness you can find inside the hoop is not about seduction. Seducing inherently involves someone outside yourself who watches and reacts to you. But to *feel sexy*, you don't need the attention of a partner or anyone other than yourself.

The divine feminine

Like happiness, true sexiness comes from *within* as you connect with what Hindus call Shakti, the divine female power. (In ancient India, the dancing temple priestesses transmitted the mystery of Shakti through their dance, using it to transmute sexual energy into spiritual bliss.) This is what distinguishes hooping from exotic and erotic dance: You do it for your own gratification rather than for someone else's.

"Hooping is the best door that has ever opened for me. When I am inside the hoop, I become a goddess. It's like being in love, completely head over heels."

—Andrea

When I hoop, I get sweaty, flushed, and tingly. But there is a bigger feeling that moves inside me—it's the feeling of being powerful. Stepping into the hoop is like stepping into lioness energy. My body feels so strong and invincible, I could roar. With the hoop between me and them, it's easier not to care what other people think and to bust loose. The masks required in the world of deadlines and skyscrapers fall away. I can be true to my beautiful self.

As I spin, I can see, hear, and smell everything at a heightened level. I become ultra aware of the parts of my body asking for nurturing. The gentle pressure of the hoop helps me surrender where I've been rigid. I yield to a celebration of all things divinely feminine—of being voluptuous, tender, and graceful. I bask, luxuriate, and blossom inside the hoop. It's this yummy space where I connect with true sexiness.

Big-Time Sensuality

A good way to get into the mood for the moves you're about to learn is to turn on some sultry music and begin warming your body up in Pump. Close your eyes— use a blindfold or Buff if you like—and run your hands over your forearms, shoulders, neck, and chest. Gently roll your head and feel the tickle of your hair as you toss it around. Rhythmically pulse your shoulders. Breathe deeply and slowly from your solar plexus, filling your lungs and expanding your rib cage.

Check your inhibitions at the door and invite your inner goddess out to play. As you practice these moves, focus on the sensation of the hoop pressing into you. Surrender to its rhythm and go with it. Make your

movements dreamy and languid—imagine you're swimming in a warm ocean at sunset or moving through molasses. Breathe deeply. Be aware of your mouth, your lips, your eyes, and your fingers. When you move onto the floor, pretend you are melting into a molten liquid state, molding your supple body to any surface you touch.

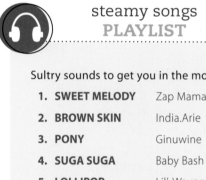

steamy songs
PLAYLIST

Sultry sounds to get you in the mood.

1. **SWEET MELODY** — Zap Mama
2. **BROWN SKIN** — India.Arie
3. **PONY** — Ginuwine
4. **SUGA SUGA** — Baby Bash
5. **LOLLIPOP** — Lil' Wayne
6. **FEELIN' LOVE** — Paula Cole
7. **TEXAS FLOOD** — Stevie Ray Vaughn
8. **THAT'S THE WAY LOVE GOES** — Janet Jackson
9. **ONE LOVE** — Sara Tavares
10. **GOODBYE SADNESS (TRISTEZA)** — Astrud Gilberto and the Walter Wanderly Trio

Electric Slide

Transition from standing to lying on the floor while swinging the hoop in WILDWEST.

variation 1

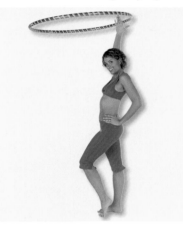

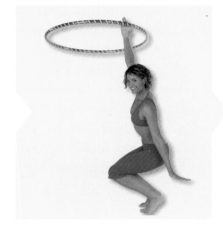

1 While spinning the hoop in WILDWEST (page 62), bend your knees slowly to lower yourself into a squatting position.

2 As you lower your butt onto the floor, slow your pace, take three full breaths in and out.

variation 2

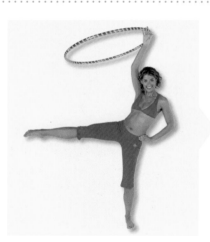

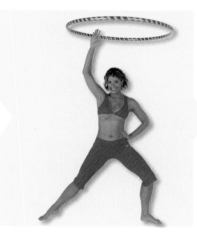

1 Get the hoop going in WILDWEST. Bend one knee slightly and lift the other leg directly up and out to the side, pointing your toe. Make sure to engage your abs.

2 Slide the extended leg to the floor into a half split, bending the knee of the standing leg lower. Keep your movements molasses-slow.

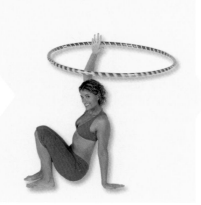

3 Support yourself with your free hand. Imagine you are sighing down onto a cushion of clouds. Lay your bent knees onto the floor like folded wings.

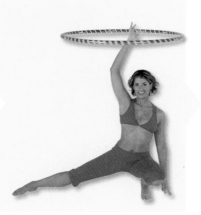

3 Continue until you can touch the floor with your free hand. Lay the outer thigh of your bent knee on the floor and shift your weight to your buns.

for either variation:

4 End in a PIN UP pose on the floor. Turn the whole length of your body to the same side as your non-hooping arm so you are lying on one side, supported by your forearm. Continue in WILDWEST. Allow the top leg to slide forward and drape gracefully over the one on the floor. Relax and luxuriate like the goddess you are!

Scissor Kick

While seated, kick forward with alternating legs while keeping the hoop in WILDWEST.

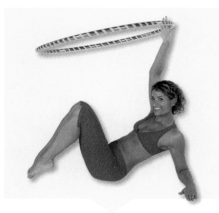

1 Sit on the floor and twirl the hoop overhead in WILDWEST. Use your other arm to stabilize yourself as you lean back and lift your feet off the floor.

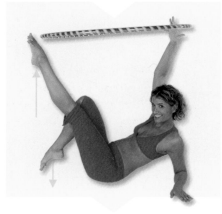

2 Engage your abs and point your toes and do a slow, graceful kick. Alternate bending and extending opposite legs. Imagine you are riding a bike, but lead with pointed toes.

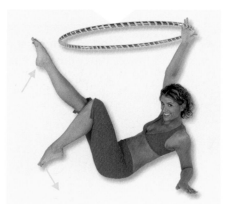

3 You may have to lean back to keep your balance between WILDWEST and kicking forward with alternating legs. Keep your back arched and abs engaged, and hold your head high.

Galaxy

Spin on your rear end as you whirl the hoop in WILDWEST.

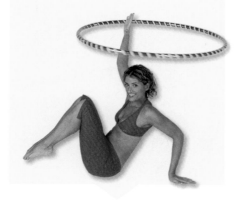

NOTE: GALAXY requires a smooth surface, like a hardwood floor.

1 While seated on the floor swinging the hoop in WILDWEST, pull your legs close to your torso, as though you're hugging your knees to your chest—but without using an arm to contain your knees. Place your other hand around back behind your hip, palm down.

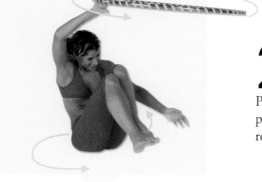

2 Powerfully push off the floor to send yourself spinning on your buns in the same direction as your hoop is rotating. Pull your legs tight to your chest with your pushing hand. The hoop should continue rotating in WILDWEST.

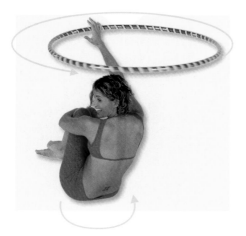

3 If you want to spin some more, place the pushing hand behind your back and push off again. Yell "Wheeeeeee!" as you go to supercharge your spin and your grin.

Lickety Split

While continuously doing WILDWEST, you'll kneel on one knee, pivot on your bottom, do a split with your legs, pivot, and end on the opposite knee.

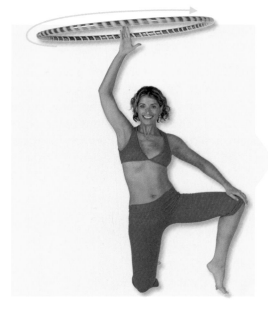

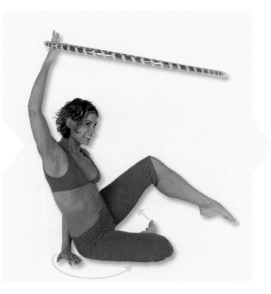

1 With one knee on the floor and the other out to your side, get the hoop into WILDWEST. Make sure the hoop is rotating toward the side of the raised knee. (If your left knee is raised, your hoop should rotate to your left.)

2 Reach behind you with your non-hoop hand and place it on the ground as you sit back on your buns. Allow the momentum of leaning back plus the WILDWEST to spin you on your butt so you end up facing the opposite direction.

a tip for triumph

▶ Let the momentum of WILDWEST roll your body through all the steps. With practice, you'll be able to connect all the parts of this wild ride fluidly.

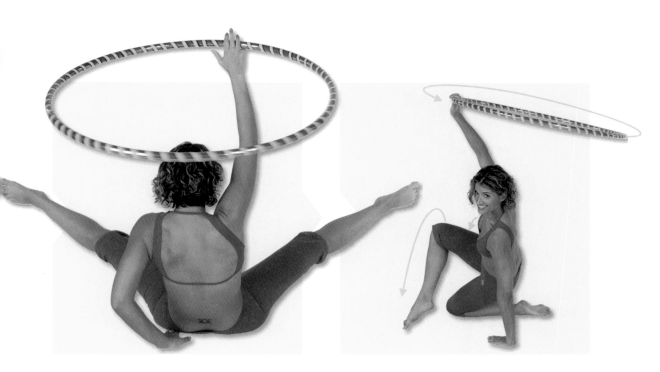

3 Extend your legs out to each side, pointing your toes. Spread your legs only as far as feels comfortable. It's okay if your knees are bent. Lean back to support your weight with your hand and to launch the turn.

4 Bring your legs together and inward to your torso, push off with your non-hoop hand.

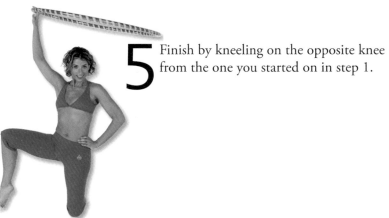

5 Finish by kneeling on the opposite knee from the one you started on in step 1.

Magic

In MAGIC, you'll spin the hoop on the floor to create a whirling globe effect.

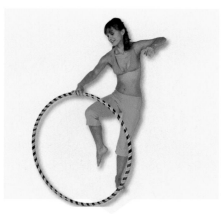

1 Place the hoop so it stands vertically on the floor, preferably on a smooth surface. Grasp your hoop at the top with one or both hands.

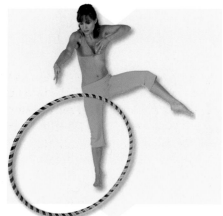

2 Twist the hoop powerfully so that it spins on its axis, independent of your hands. Groove alongside your spinning hoop like it's your dance partner! Extend your arms toward it as if you're "conjuring" its motion.

3 As the hoop begins to slow and wobble, grasp it at the top and quickly retwist it in the same or opposite direction to spin onward. This is great for improving hand-eye coordination.

Lakshmi

While the hoop balances atop your head, slowly and meditatively move the rest of your body.

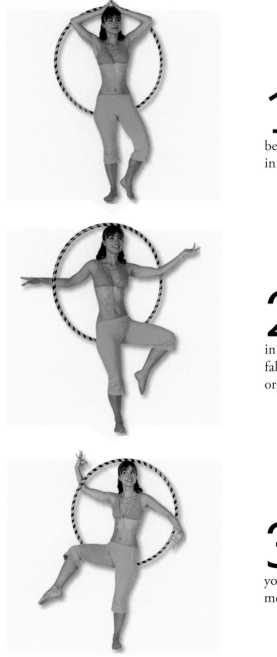

1 Find the spot on your head with the best balance. Place the hoop on top of your head so the opening of the hoop is behind you. If the hoop won't stay put, hold it in place with both hands in a prayer pose.

2 With your shoulders back and your chest open, lift one leg, bending the knee and moving it through space in slow motion, as in tai chi. If the hoop falls, replace it. Keep your limbs flowing organically.

3 Combine languid shoulder and torso movement. If you can keep the hoop aloft without one or both hands, move your arms too. This is great for balance and meditation.

Fantasy

Holding the hoop around you on a horizontal plane, raise and lower it while turning to give the illusion that the hoop is levitating.

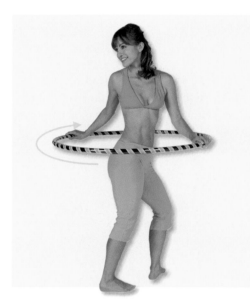

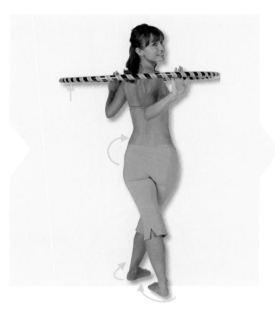

1 Stand in the center of the hoop and hold it around you. Grip with both hands, palms down, and with your thumbs on the inside of the hoop. Keep it flat, on the horizontal plane, at all times.

2 Pivot or take steps to turn your body. The hoop is naturally turning with you, held fast in the same grip, with you as its center. Your feet never stop moving in FANTASY, so take a break at any point if you feel dizzy.

challenge yourself!

▶ Use just *one* hand to raise and lower the hoop. You'll need to grip the hoop tightly, yet loosen your grip as the hoop changes levels, all the while keeping it on the horizontal plane. This takes a lot of wrist strength. Alternate hands, practice in small doses, and use a lightweight hoop.

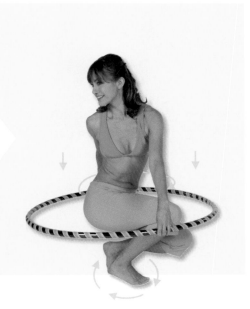

DANCE-IFY IT

Coil your spine by looking back over your shoulder at your buns. This creates a beautiful S shape and stretches your vertebrae.

3 Begin lifting the hoop upward in slow motion. As you raise it, your grip should loosen so your palms slide to the inside. Go up on tiptoes, extending your arms up as high as possible, allowing your grip to shift again to the hoop's underside.

4 Now lower your body and the hoop slowly, while continuing to turn your body. As you go lower, your palms will slide around to the top of the hoop. Take long, relaxed breaths to slow your movements. The hoop should appear to be levitating around you.

• Continue raising and lowering the hoop with fluid movements. Imagine you are a whirling dervish, spinning perfectly around a center point.

Tantric Awakenings

THREE YEARS BEFORE I DISCOVERED HOOPING, I had a major Kundalini awakening. That's when the energy at the base of your spine, feminine/Shakti, moves upward and merges with the crown chakra, masculine/Shiva. In Eastern yogic traditions, a magical coiled serpent lies dormant at the base of the spine, awaiting stimulation. When this serpent is roused, it rises up the spine to the head, causing an orgasmic sense of connection and enlightenment.

So I recognized the sensation when it happened in hoop class. We were learning to turn within the hoop, and as I began to spin around, "I" disappeared, and what was left of me was a blissful, ecstatic feeling of expansion.

I realized that hooping mimics a lot of what went on during my Kundalini awakening. As the hoop rolls around your hips, it activates your second chakra, the sexual and creative center. When you undulate to move the hoop up your spine and circle it around your chest, it opens your heart center. The spiraling movement of the hoop up the torso evokes the serpent's rising and uncoiling and releases a blast of energy. Hooping is like shaking a rattle that activates Shakti. If you add turns, you accelerate the spinning of the chakra system.

This creates a spiritual opening in which the body can receive more light (information) and inspiration.

I now incorporate hooping into my work as a tantric healer and teacher. Because the hoop spends much of its time spinning around the Sacral chakra, which is connected to sensuality and sexuality, hooping heightens awareness in these areas.

I believe sexual energy is the creative force of the universe. It is my passion to unlock that wisdom in my clients' bodies. The hoop is a wonderful tool for this.

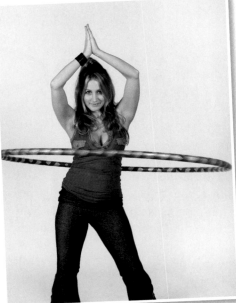

Name: Shari
Occupation: Tantric Healer

Hooping and Sexual Vibrance

MARIA MUSCARELLA, A NURSE WHO SPECIALIZES in women's health, has witnessed significant impacts on her clients' reproductive systems and sex drive from hooping. "By increasing movement in the pelvis, you are increasing the flow of blood, energy/chi, and nerve conduction. How could that not have a positive effect? Where there is more blood and energy, the cells will be more nourished and functional," she says. And by *functional*, she means in bed. She recommends hooping to clients who experience "stagnation in their pelvic region" or who feel disconnected from that part of their bodies.

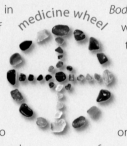

medicine wheel

DR. CHRISTIANE NORTHRUP IS A MIND-BODY health pioneer who spent twenty years practicing obstetrics and gynecology. In her book *Women's Bodies, Women's Wisdom* she writes: "Women who have healthy, strong pelvic muscles . . . tend to have more fulfilling sexual functioning with better pelvic blood flow, better vaginal lubrication, and stronger orgasms." Hooping builds those pelvic muscles. As Northrup, who hoops herself, says: "I recommend moving your hips with a Hula Hoop for your circulatory health, for weight loss, for just plain fun and all-around health."

Spiraling Energy

By now you know: Hooping moves stuff around. The hoop massages acupressure points and powers your circulation. Your blood flows more vigorously and your lymph is pumped along. Your mood is lifted and your life force, or chi, is mobilized.

Some cultures believe that energy moves through seven centers positioned between the tailbone and the crown of the head. These are known as the *chakras,* which is a Sanskrit term meaning circles or wheels. Like hoops, chakras spin as they convey energy. Each one represents a different quality (like purification or kindness) and connects to different organs and endocrine glands in the body. When energy cycles through them freely and in balance, your body-mind-spirit stays healthy—when stagnation occurs, physical or emotional problems arise.

Like yoga, hooping can assist the flow of energy. The hoop rolls directly over some chakras while the other chakras are affected by the spinning and movement itself. The act of spiraling the hoop from the knees, up the torso, over the head in your hand, then back down your body again incites the flow of energy through all seven centers.

The Chakras: Spinning Wheels of Energy

Use this chart to identify the chakra responsible for an area or quality of your life that you want to address. I've linked each chakra to specific moves so you can guide your hooping practice to impact those areas directly. Dedicate time to practicing certain moves with the intent of channeling specific energy, and see what happens. You just might be surprised at the effects.

ROOT CHAKRA

TAKING RESPONSIBILITY FOR YOU

Survival • Integrity • Grounding • Responsibility • Nourishment • Earth • Rooted • Solid • Gravity • Primal • Safe • Familiar • Stillness • Heavy • Basic Needs Met • Stability • Accepting the Body

The root chakra is found at the base of the spine and is about earthy foundations. Use BOOTY BLITZ to stimulate this area, GARTER to activate your legs, and floor moves like SCISSOR KICK to feel connected to the earth. You also access this chakra by deliberately making your movements very grounded while hooping.

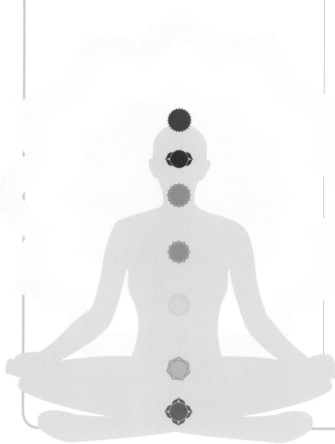

SACRAL CHAKRA

OWNING YOUR DIVINE BEAUTY

Pleasure • Sensuality • Sexuality • Abundance • Emotions • Flowing • Sweetness • Desire • Nurturing • Liquid • Intimacy • Touching

The sacral chakra is in the abdomen, lower back, and sexual organs. You energize this chakra by spinning the hoop around your core—as in PUMP, BOOTY BLITZ, LIMBO, or SLINKY. Sassy moves like PIN UP, BLING, and BUN help you connect with the flirtatious, sensual energy of this area.

SOLAR PLEXUS CHAKRA

EMPOWERING YOUR SELF

Fire • Drive • Determination • Focus
• Forceful • Metabolism • Directing
• Powerful • Energizing • Mobilizing
• Will • Transforming • Control • Individuality

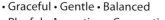

The solar plexus chakra is associated with the power of your will and individuality. Play with moves like Barrel Roll, Warrior, Spunk, or Pulse to channel its energy.

HEART CHAKRA

WELCOMING YOUR INNER CHILD

Loving • Open • Giving • Worthy
• Graceful • Gentle • Balanced
• Playful • Accepting • Connecting
• Peaceful • Joyous • Humorous
• Lighthearted • Healing • Compassionate

The heart chakra can be activated by hooping with friends, playing, and laughing. Whoopee, Sparkle, and Galaxy invoke the playful energy. Moves like Disco and Snake ask you to directly open your heart.

THROAT CHAKRA

WALKING YOUR TALK

Vibrating • Expressing • Vocalizing
• Communicating • Transmitting
• Expanding • Purifying • Creating
Meaning • Telepathic • Resonance

The throat chakra is about vocalizing, owning your truth, and sharing it with the world. You can access it by doing Pearl or adding your voice to specific hooping moves as I've suggested.

THIRD-EYE CHAKRA

AWAKENING YOUR INTUITION

Color • Psychic • Imagining
• Visualizing • Perceiving
• Dreams • Memory • All-Seeing
• All-Knowing • Light-filled • Clairvoyance
• Space/Time Awareness

The third-eye chakra is related to the act of seeing, both physically and intuitively. Explore this energy by hooping blindfolded. Or use the rich symbolism of moves like Magic or Portal to access the transcendent energy of the third eye.

CROWN CHAKRA

CONNECTING TO ONE-NESS

Understanding • Enlightenment
• Beliefs • Cosmic Consciousness
• Information • Thoughts • Knowing • Meditation
• Channeling • Transcendence

The crown chakra is our connection to a vast, timeless place of all-knowing. Call forth this energy through moves that involve sustained whirling like Fantasy and Disco, as well as through moves that are meditative, like Lakshmi or the simple, blissful Pump.

THE MOVES

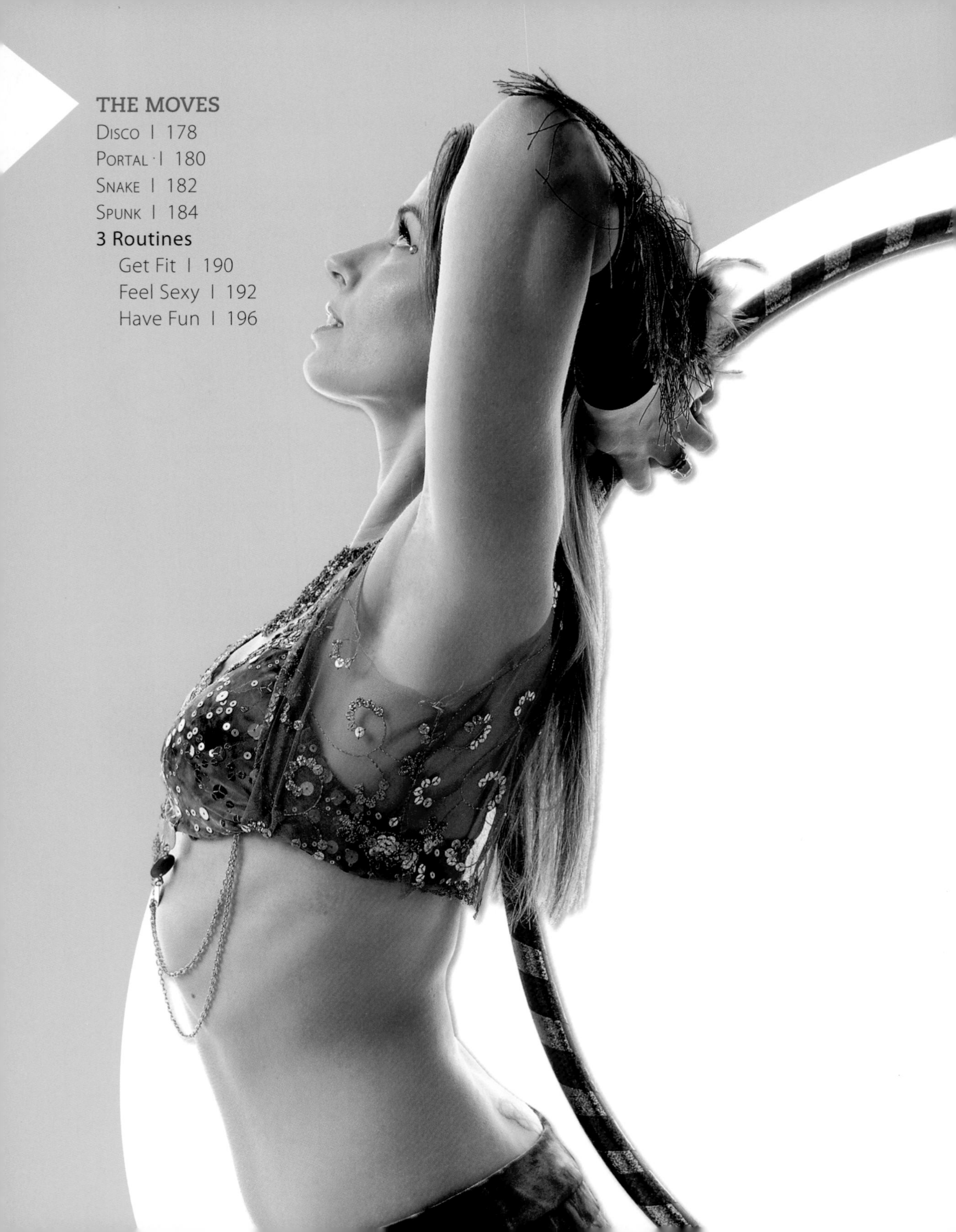

The Pinnacle & Beyond

PRACTICE & ROUTINES

So, you've been hooping for a while now—how do you feel? Can you feel the increased strength in your abs? Are you energized? Are you more aware of your body? What about your mood? Do you feel proud of your hooping accomplishments? Exhilarated to have achieved orbit and learned some new moves? Do you wake up looking forward to the day's hooping session? Have you been telling everyone in your life about your new passion?

If your answer to these questions is YES, congratulations! You can officially call yourself a *hooper,* and join the tens of thousands of us who rely on our hoops for health, fitness, happiness, and sanity.

Every hooper is created equal. True, some of us have grooved for years as opposed to weeks or months, yet your individuality shines through your hoop and your dance. Some people are more flexible, some have cleaner moves, some are more agile, more expressive, more playful, or more linear . . . there's an amazing diversity! A beginner often has just as much to teach an advanced hooper as the other way around. A fresh-eyed newbie can see possibilities for the hoop without old habits getting in the way.

Of course, there is one key difference between you and a veteran hooper, and that's the amount of practice time you've put in. Most hoop moves aren't like sit-ups or leg lifts—exercises you only need to see once to do on your own. They require a little more practice. It takes time to evolve from spinning to soaring.

FOUR STAGES OF HOOPDANCE

1. BLISS

As in—"Ignorance is . . ." You're totally caught up in the thrill of the hoop circling your waist and in the excitement of something new and playful. It's a time of whirling wonder, free of any need to achieve or aspire to more. You bask in the stillness of the center while the repetitive motion calms your mind.

2. INSPIRATION

As in—Breathe it in. There's a whole world of hooping out there to discover: tricks and skills, celebrities and teachers, video channels, workshops, and conventions! You have to keep breathing and not get ahead of yourself. Persistence is power.

3. CONNECTION

An *aha!* moment. Moves "click" and things fall into place. You gain speed, agility, and precision. You begin to link moves and add personal flair. Your practice becomes an end in itself, instead of a path to somewhere. Stay humble and receptive.

4. FLOW

Your body knows the way. You don't need your brain to explain how to do a move, or what comes next in your dance. The music, your hoop, and you have the ease of old friends. Unfettered creativity explodes in new combinations and "signature" phrases of movement that are yours alone. The challenge is to hold on to a "beginner's mind" and keep learning and growing.

The four stages are cyclical, not linear, which might mean you progress

BLISS INSPIRATION

FLOW CONNECTION

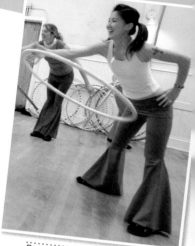

Practice, practice, practice!

from Flow to Bliss, or are in Inspiration and Connection at the same time. Maybe you're in Flow with a move like PUMP, and still in the Inspiration phase while practicing the BARREL ROLL or LIBRA.

Resolutions for Revolutions

To master the moves and create flow in your hoopdance, you need to practice. And then practice some more. Classes and hoopgroups can open your eyes to new possibilities, yet they are no substitute for regular personal practice time—time alone with your hoop. Your hoop is the purest teacher you can find!

And since it's just you, you can arrange your practice time to suit your own schedule. Find a time and space to be undisturbed by others, including your kids. Banish the BlackBerry or turn a blind eye to your iPhone. Welcome the undistracted focus on YOU. I like to think that my personal practice time requires *blissipline,* a version of discipline in which I'm both my own tough-love drill sergeant and euphoric cheerleader.

To maintain your practice, it may help to write down a set of goals—along with how and when you'll reach them. Putting it in writing means a real commitment, not just wishful thinking. One goal could be mastering one of the three additional routines you'll find beginning on page 189.

Then dream up rewards and give them to yourself—not just for mastering a move, but for steps along the way. It might be a handful of strawberries, a soak in a hot tub, a new hoop, or tickets to Cirque du Soleil. You deserve it!

If you can show up for your hoop, you can show up for other things in your life. Think of approaching your hoop practice as a form of "soul tending"—an opportunity to restore and rejuvenate yourself. You can go to your hoop if you feel down or discouraged, as a place to heal. If you feel disconnected and alone, the hoop can remind you how cosmically connected you are. Take your practice as deep as you feel you need it.

Now, as you learn the four final fabulous moves—DISCO, PORTAL, SNAKE, and SPUNK— be patient with yourself. Many people require *months* of practice before they achieve graceful execution of these more advanced moves, so keep the faith! And go ahead and giggle. A sense of humor is invaluable in meeting the challenges here.

Disco

The hoop rests against your chest, stationary in the horizontal plane, as you turn your body. The momentum of your spinning keeps the hoop aloft and as the chest expands to hold the hoop, the heart opens.

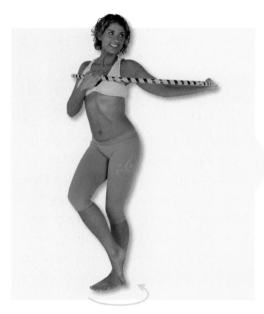

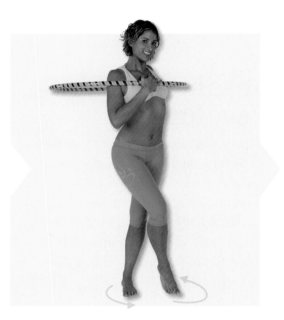

1 Stand inside the hoop, pressing it to your sternum with one hand. Support the opposite edge of the hoop behind you, extending your arm fully. Keep the hoop as horizontal as possible.

2 Take steps to turn your body in a circle. By holding the hoop in place, you can keep your footwork slow and still enjoy the feel of the move. This is a great way to do this move if you're prone to dizziness.

a tip for triumph

▶ Begin by practicing your spin without the hoop. Use tape to mark a spot on the floor, and stay centered on it as you take lightning-fast steps— almost a run while pivoting, like a whirling dervish— to turn your body in a tight circle.

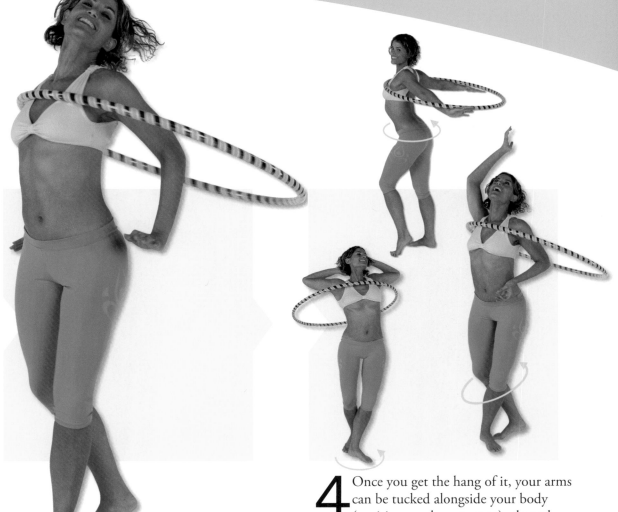

3 Feel when your body is spinning fast enough that you can let go of the hoop and rely on momentum to keep it in place, "hanging" freely on the horizontal plane. Expand your chest by arching your back. Push out against the hoop to keep it aloft.

4 Once you get the hang of it, your arms can be tucked alongside your body (envision an elegant crane), clasped behind your head, or extended behind you. Envision yourself as a shining star whirling through the cosmos, perfectly balanced.

• If you feel the hoop slipping down your chest, speed up your footwork or support the hoop with your arms until you feel it being carried by your momentum once more.

Portal

The hoop spins on the vertical plane around a stationary point, creating the illusion that it is suspended in midair. It is mesmerizing to behold! Think magical mirrors and passages into another realm . . .

NOTE: Use a lightweight hoop to prevent strain on your hands.

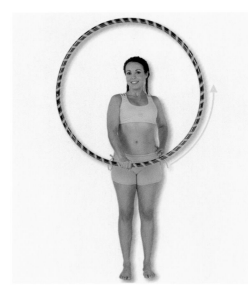

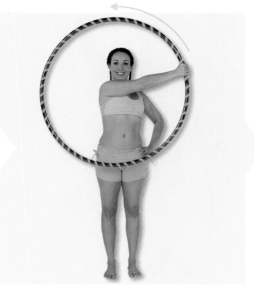

1 To begin, hold the hoop on the vertical plane in front of you, using your right hand. Grip the hoop at the bottom with your palm facing the ground and your arm extended downward.

2 From this position, slowly move your hand clockwise around the "clock," taking the hoop with it (do not release or switch the grip). Your right hand is now palm up on the inside of the hoop.

3 At the top, switch hands. Place your left hand on the hoop beside your right, palms up, pinky to pinky. Release your right hand.

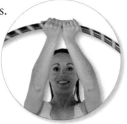

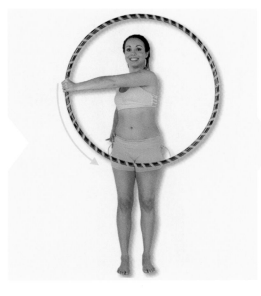

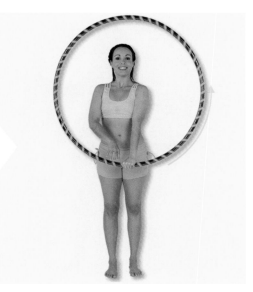

4 With your left hand, slowly move around the clock back down to 6 o'clock, grasping the hoop continuously.

5 At 6 o'clock your left hand should be facing the ground, as at the beginning. Again grasp the hoop with your right hand. Release your left hand and move back up to 12 o'clock.

a tip for triumph

▶ With the help of a mirror, or by "soft focusing" your eyes, look at where the top of the hoop is in relation to other visual reference points, such as how far it is above (or below) the top of your head. You want the hoop to stay in this exact spot the whole time you are doing PORTAL. Notice where on the clock you need to adjust the extension of your arm to keep the hoop "suspended" in its spot.

Snake

In this surefire "wow"-inducing move, the hoop revolves around your upper arms and chest on the horizontal plane. To master SNAKE, constantly turn in the same direction as the hoop.

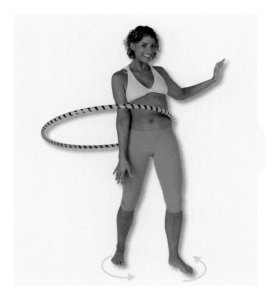

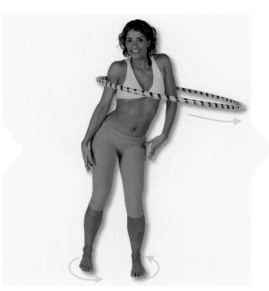

1 Get the hoop in PUMP and start turning. Extend one arm inside the hoop as in SLINKY (page 76), but instead of pulling it back out, keep that arm pressed against your body and continue to PUMP.

2 Slip the other arm in and using the surface of your arms (ideally your biceps) nudge the hoop up incrementally to just above your breasts. To achieve this, some people visualize using their arms like spoons to "stir" the area inside the hoop. Try to relax your shoulders and elbows and remember to breathe.

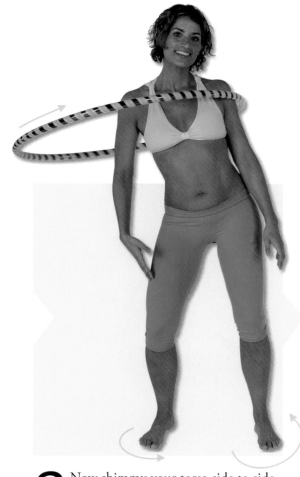

3 Now shimmy your torso side to side (as opposed to forward and back) while still turning. Leading with your elbows and using the surface of your triceps (as if you were elbowing someone out of the way), push out and diagonally into the hoop whenever you feel it make contact. Bare arms make this easier.

4 As much as you can, exert pressure all the way around inside the hoop, using your upper arms, bringing your chest diagonally forward to meet the hoop, and pushing diagonally back with your upper back. Envision the spinal spiraling of a cobra. Keep turning and breathing!

a tip for triumph

▶ If the hoop drops, capture it in PUMP by resuming the forward-back motion of your hips. When you are ready, insert your arms again, nudge the hoop up, and continue the side-to-side/diagonal pulsation in your upper body.

Spunk

Rotate the hoop around your legs on the horizontal plane while turning. There is no way to do SPUNK *slowly—you must invest yourself 110 percent!*

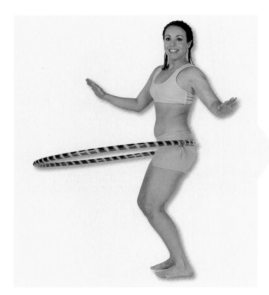

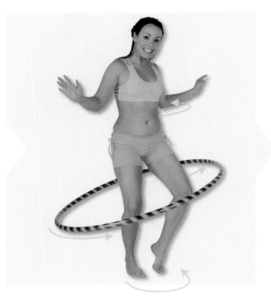

1 Start in BOOTY BLITZ (page 42) while turning in the same direction as the hoop's rotation. Slow down the motion of your hips so that the hoop drops below your buttocks. As soon as it reaches your thighs, slightly raise one knee by going up on your toes. (Your left knee if you're hooping to the left, or your right if you're hooping to the right.) This is your "swivel leg."

2 As the hoop rolls over the thigh of your swivel leg, pivot on its toe to swing the leg outward into the hoop, pushing the hoop along.

The swivel leg needs to swing rapidly side to side to push the hoop along. To swing it more easily, pivot on your toes and turn your body continuously, using your standing leg to push off.

a tip for triumph

▶ Make SPUNK easier by turning continuously inside the hoop in the direction of its rotation. Focusing on your CONTACT POINTS can also help: One is roughly on the front of your thigh (your left thigh, if your INFLOW is to the left) and the other is on the back of your opposite thigh.

3 As soon as the hoop rolls over your back thigh, swing the swivel leg back in so it's pressed against the other leg. It may help to visualize your swivel leg as the flapping wing of a bird.

4 Repeat steps 3 and 4 over and over as a rapid-fire suite of movements. You will be constantly moving—turning your body and pushing with your thighs. Keep breathing!

• Aim to keep the hoop on the fleshy part of your thighs so that it is comfortable and fun. Your hoop will undoubtedly clatter to the floor at first, but keep your spirits high.

Hooping the Light Fantastic

"What we need are more people who specialize in the impossible."

—*Theodore Roethke, poet*

Over time, as you continue hooping, you may find yourself becoming lighter. Heaviness and "baggage," both physical and emotional, can disappear. You may notice more ease, flow, and joyfulness in your thoughts. Perhaps your steps will have more spring and bounce. Your heart may feel more open and carefree. Your skin may even look more radiant and youthful (profuse sweating does that!). But consider that there may be some other alchemy at work.

Ancient Indian Buddhists believed that all reality was created by light. They believed time is moving through the Gold, Silver, Bronze, and Iron Ages. In other words, humanity has been progressively moving from beauty and light into dimmer times of chaos. But there is hope. Humanity's salvation lies with the Goddess Kali's dance of transformation, which draws out negative energy and changes it into love. Her sacred dance is supposed to purify the earth and restore us to an age of beauty, peace, and radiance.

This myth speaks to me personally, to my ability to dance through negative emotion or physical discomfort and to radiate healing light from my heart. Just maybe, hoopdance can accelerate communication, healing, and peace. Just maybe, the hoop helps you channel the divine. Step in, give it a whirl, and see what happens!

NO EXCUSES

Excuses, excuses—I've heard them all before. Instead of seeing these things as obstacles to your practice, reframe them as opportunities.

SPACE. Think you don't have enough of it? I often practice in a five-by-six-foot spot in my living room, between the TV, heater, and sofa. The coffee table is on casters, so it rolls out of the way. I set up a long mirror against one wall and use it to spot my posture. There's a ceiling fan with a glass bulb cover, and yes, I have to watch out for it—and the mirror.

View space constrictions as opportunities to develop control, precision, and spatial awareness. Be creative, selecting more contained movements to practice (for example, PUMP, PORTAL, or MAGIC) and keeping the others for outdoor practice.

Make your space hoop-friendly: Banish children and pets. Remove glass of any kind, turning monitors and screens to face away from you if possible. Although a hoop will almost never break a standard window, cover old, thin panes with drapes. Avoid vertical moves such as WARRIOR near overhead light fixtures. And don't hoop blindfolded.

PLATEAU. This is a natural part of the learning process. Jump-start your enthusiasm if it starts to wane, by, for example, watching hooping videos at sites like YouTube, or by playing with hoops of different sizes. Sometimes some fresh tunes are all you need to get your hoop on again. Grab your Buff for a tantalizing sightless challenge, or pick a new focus for your practice, like hooping in your OUTFLOW or deepening your breath.

MOOD. Instead of thinking you need to be in a certain mood to practice, tell yourself that practice is a path to the mood you want to feel. If you've had a tough day or feel overwhelmed with how much you've got to do, think again about hooping. Ride out the rough spot in your hoop and you may find yourself sailing into new insights or breakthroughs.

INJURY. If you have a localized injury, it might be an opportunity to focus on very specific drills and isolations that you don't normally do. For example, an ankle injury could creatively restrict you to focus on PORTAL. A wrist injury might be an invitation to keep the hoop on your core for the entire practice session. Remain open to alternative possibilities.

TIME. There are 1,440 minutes in every day . . . use just twenty of those to get your groove on! Set the kitchen timer for twenty minutes just a couple days a week. You may find yourself continuing to hoop past the buzzer. Ease may get the better of your resistance! Remember that claiming some special time for you each day is a gift to yourself.

Pay attention to the stories you tell yourself and notice when you fall into self-criticism and judgment. Dismiss thoughts that begin with "I should have . . . ," "I wish that . . . ," "If only . . . , " "I can't . . . " A halfway completed practice session is a glass half-full. And a FULL session is a glass full of champagne: Toast yourself!

HoopGirl's Last Word

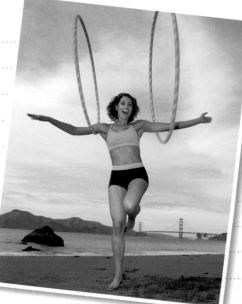

Actually, it's two words: THANK YOU. Whatever brought you here, I want to thank you for taking the time to whirl with me and discover the joys of hooping.

As the vibrant, miraculous heroine or hero of your own journey, remember to keep saying, "Yes I can!" to your hoop and to your life. Remember to keep your childlike sense of wonder and playfulness. Encourage those around you who are inspired by your craft with generous assistance. Indulge in pleasure, fun, and delightful hooping adventures. Anticipate miracles unfolding through your practice!

And no matter what, keep hooping. Hoop during lunch breaks. Hoop in the morning. Hoop in the park. Hoop on your roof. Just keep coming home to your hoop. Every social interaction is an opportunity to move with grace, flow, ease, and confidence—as you do in the hoop. Bring your light as a hooper to your every appearance. Whether it's in front of your bosses, your family, or friends. Shine in celebration of being alive.

Your hoop is a training wheel that can help you rise to your highest potential in all spheres of your life. Thank you, again, for allowing me to introduce it to you.

XOXO,
Christabel

3 Routines

GET FIT, FEEL SEXY, HAVE FUN

Once you have practiced all the moves, put them together into routines! You can combine moves in any way that creates a sense of flow for you. Here are three sets of combinations to get you started, each with a different "feel."

Some of the transitions from one move to another are simple and obvious, while others will require your creativity and finesse. Give them a whirl, then mix and match moves to create your very own combinations.

Get Fit

A 10-Move Routine to build strength, muscle, and endurance

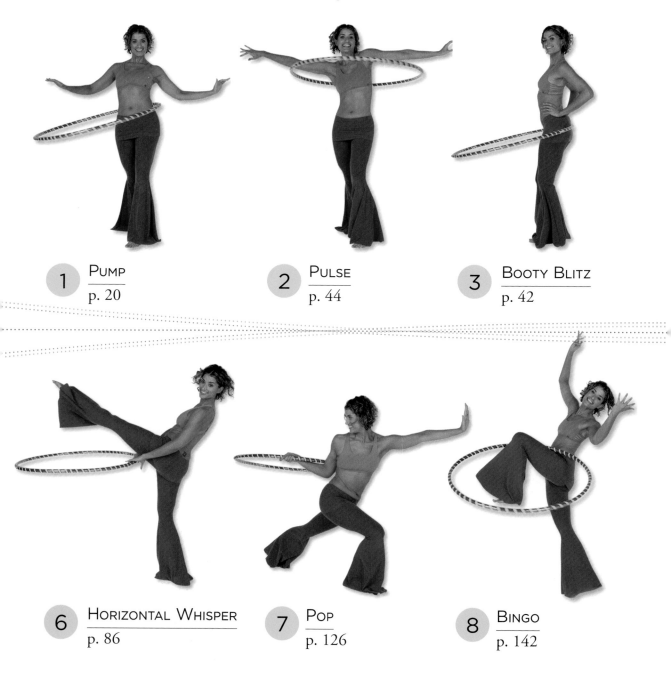

1 PUMP
p. 20

2 PULSE
p. 44

3 BOOTY BLITZ
p. 42

6 HORIZONTAL WHISPER
p. 86

7 POP
p. 126

8 BINGO
p. 142

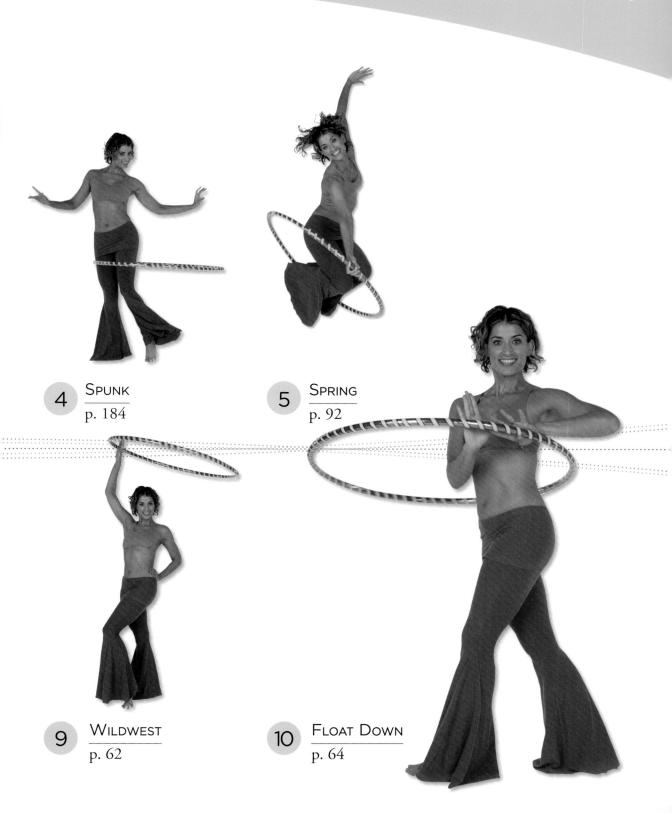

4 SPUNK
p. 184

5 SPRING
p. 92

9 WILDWEST
p. 62

10 FLOAT DOWN
p. 64

Feel Sexy

15-Move Routine to connect with your sensual inner Goddess

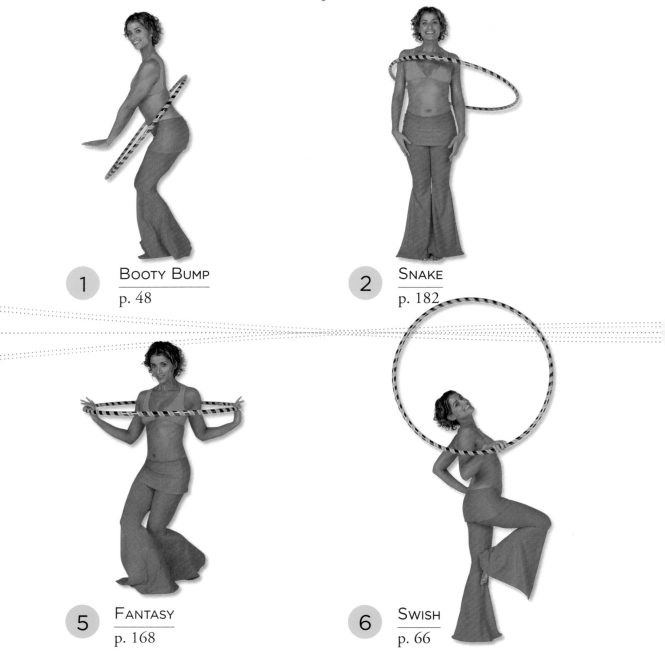

1 — BOOTY BUMP
p. 48

2 — SNAKE
p. 182

5 — FANTASY
p. 168

6 — SWISH
p. 66

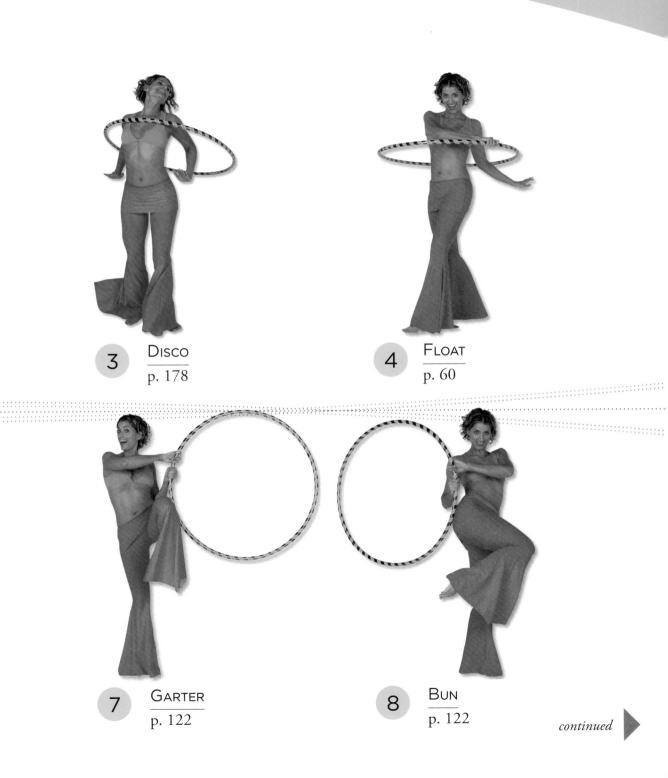

3 · DISCO
p. 178

4 · FLOAT
p. 60

7 · GARTER
p. 122

8 · BUN
p. 122

continued

▶ Feel Sexy (continued)

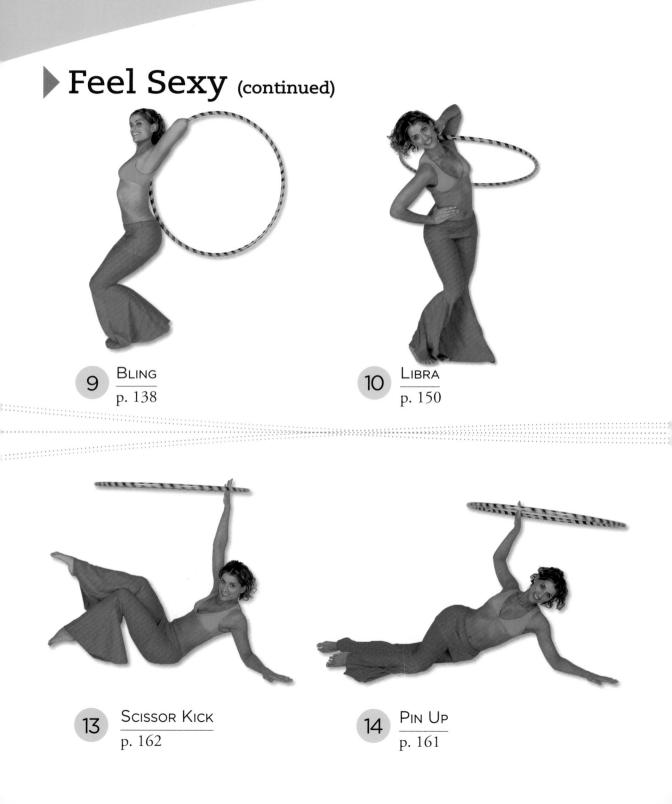

9 Bling
p. 138

10 Libra
p. 150

13 Scissor Kick
p. 162

14 Pin Up
p. 161

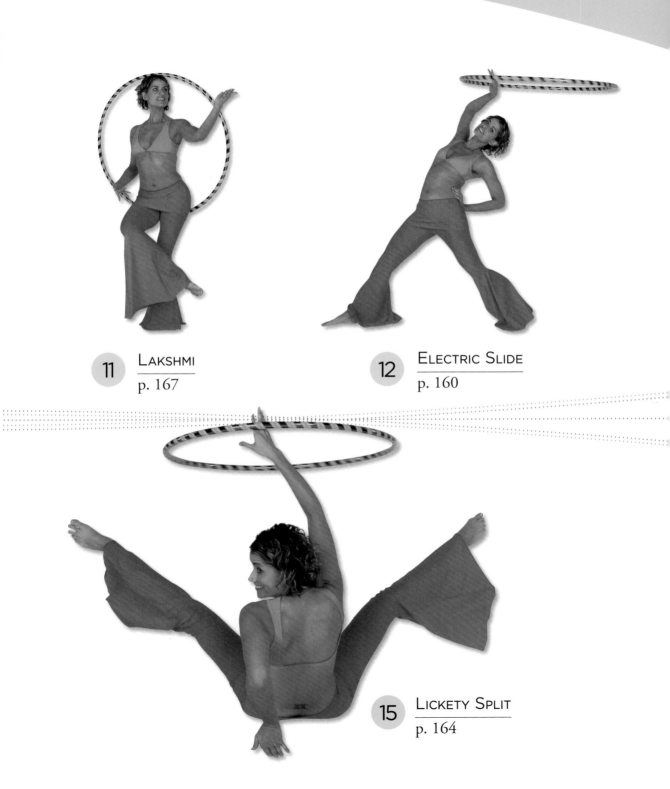

Have Fun

30-Move Routine to feel like a kid again

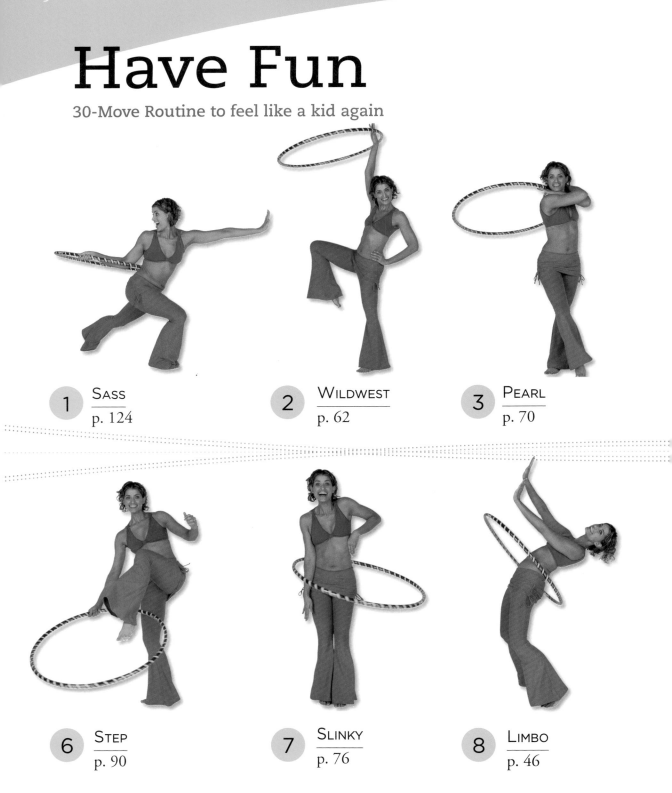

1 SASS
   p. 124

2 WILDWEST
   p. 62

3 PEARL
   p. 70

6 STEP
   p. 90

7 SLINKY
   p. 76

8 LIMBO
   p. 46

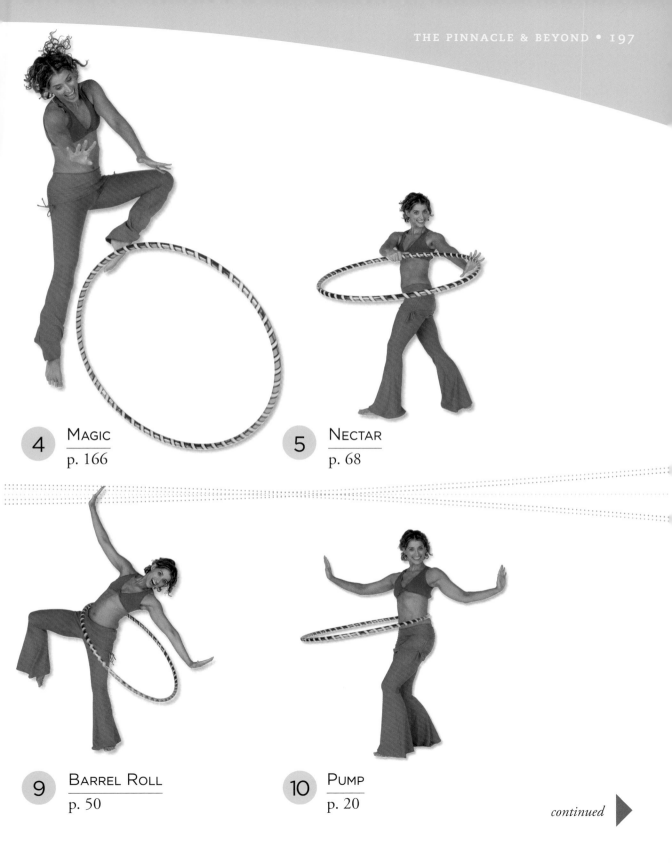

4   MAGIC
p. 166

5   NECTAR
p. 68

9   BARREL ROLL
p. 50

10   PUMP
p. 20

continued ▶

▶ Have Fun (continued)

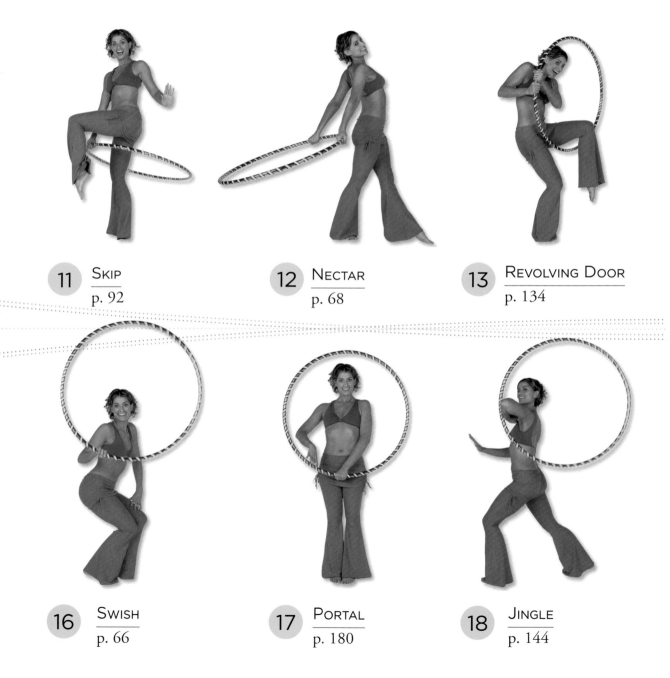

| 11 | SKIP p. 92 | 12 | NECTAR p. 68 | 13 | REVOLVING DOOR p. 134 |

| 16 | SWISH p. 66 | 17 | PORTAL p. 180 | 18 | JINGLE p. 144 |

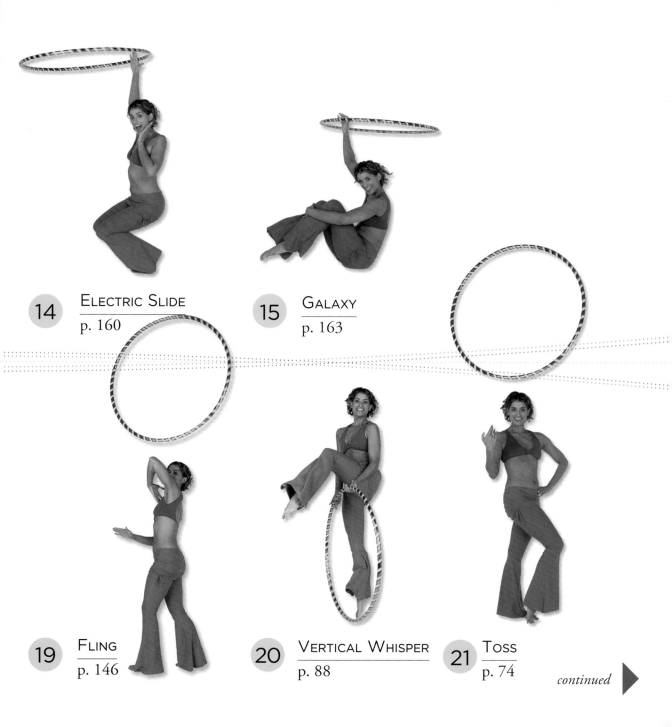

14 ELECTRIC SLIDE
p. 160

15 GALAXY
p. 163

19 FLING
p. 146

20 VERTICAL WHISPER
p. 88

21 TOSS
p. 74

continued ▶

▶ Have Fun (continued)

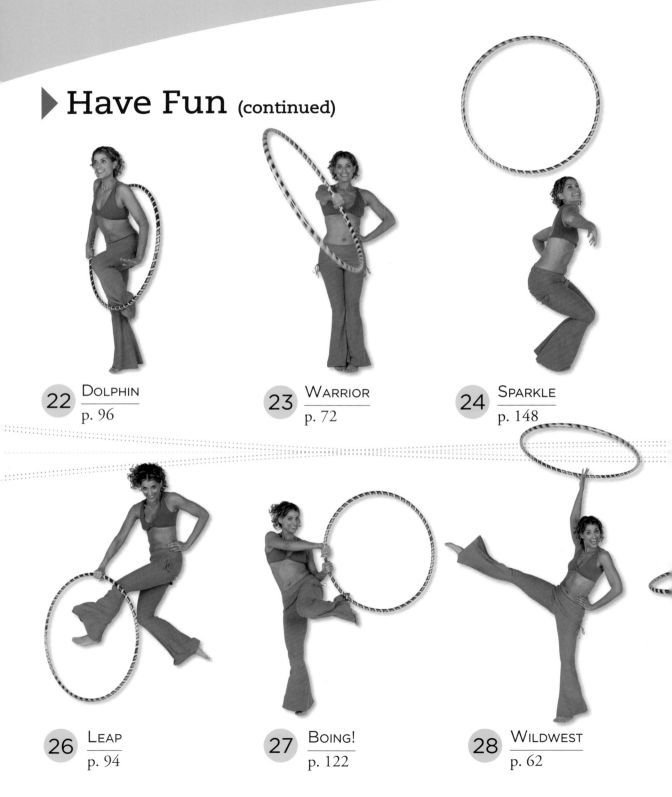

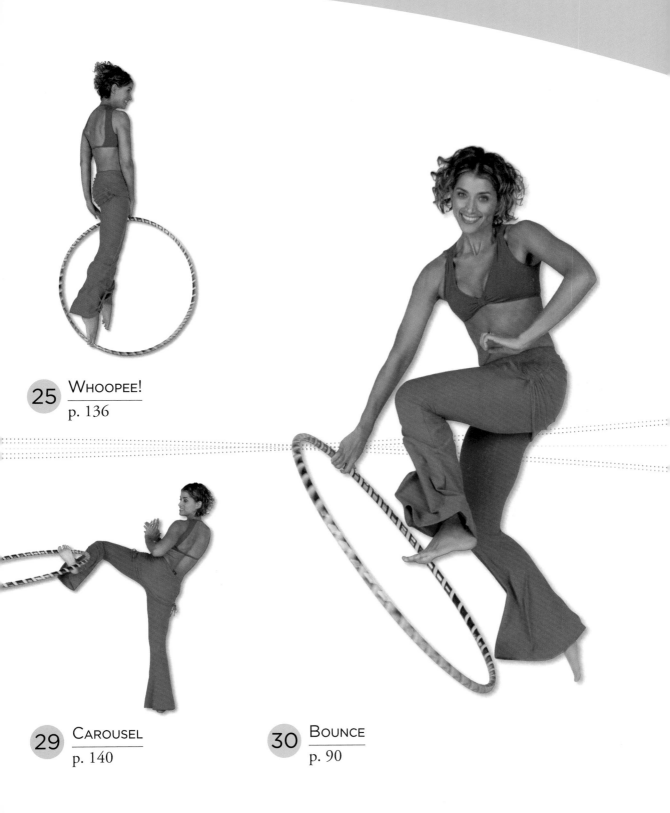

25 <u>WHOOPEE!</u>
p. 136

29 <u>CAROUSEL</u>
p. 140

30 <u>BOUNCE</u>
p. 90

APPENDIX I

Resources

HoopGirl sells a variety of professional hoops in different weights and sizes (Power, Energy, Action, Ultra, Zip and Zoom, and special-edition hoops), instructional DVDs, clothing, buffs and other hooping lifestyle products. There you can also get information about Levels 1–3 HoopGirl Teacher Certification programs, an international licensed teacher directory, classes, performances, and trainings by the HoopGirl Allstars, and annual retreats. Go to www.HoopGirl.com.

HOOP EVENTS

www.worldhoopday.com
www.hoopcampretreats.com
www.hoopconvergence.com
www.burningman.com

ONLINE HOOP RESOURCES AND DISCUSSION GROUPS

www.hooping.org
www.hoopuniversity.com
hoopgoddess.wordpress.com
www.hooping.tribe.net
www.hoopingvideos.tribe.net
www.HoopingLife.com

HOOP CLOTHING

www.hoopclothes.com
www.shaktidancewear.com
www.annieland.net

HOOP MUSIC

www.djkramer.com
www.thefitnessdj.com
www.opsinamusic.com
www.thedeependcamp.com
www.pandora.com
www.beatport.com

CHRISTABEL'S HOOPING NETWORK

www.bodyhoops.com
www.hoopnotica.com
www.hooppath.com
www.hooprevolution.com
www.hoopshine.com
www.isopop.com
www.sharnarose.co.uk
www.spiralhoopdance.com

CONNECT TO HOOPGIRL

www.twitter.com/hoopgirl
www.myspace.com/hoopgirlsuperstar
www.hoopgirl.tribe.net
www.facebook.com (HoopGirl Fans Unite)

APPENDIX II

Hooping & the Raw:
Nutritional Notes from Christabel

People are always asking me what I eat. And because I frequently write about a new smoothie or supplement on Twitter or Facebook, I get loads of e-mails asking about nutritional advice.

First, let me be clear, I am not a purist. I get cravings for chocolate and popcorn and pizza just like everyone else. But what I try to do is find whole food replacements for processed foods, and I buy organic as much as possible. If I'm feeling hungry, I ask myself, "What am I craving?" and I eat something to meet that need specifically. For example, when I crave pasta, I'll go for sprouted brown rice or quinoa. If I need something that feels heavy, I'll have a piece of avocado or organic raw almond butter slathered on wheat toast. If I want something sweet, I'll have fruit or a smoothie. When I crave meat, I'll have sushi, free-range, organic chicken, wild fish, or beef. Overall, I try to strike a balance by eating about 50 percent raw veggies and fruits and 50 percent whole grains, nuts, and proteins.

What I put into my body makes a tremendous difference in my hooping. I've always tried to eat healthfully, but the stamina and endurance I require for high-energy hoopdance has heightened my

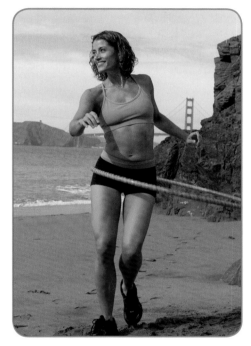

awareness even further. Café Gratitude, a raw foods restaurant in San Francisco, and Victoria Boutenko's book *Green for Life* have made a huge impact on me, inspiring me to add blended green drinks to my daily health regimen. Boutenko's research shows that raw foods contain more nutrients than processed foods, and that the more raw, organic green foods you eat, the more you shift your body's pH from acid to alkaline. The Nobel Prize–winning scientist, Otto

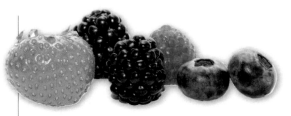

Warburg, proved that cancer thrives in acidic conditions. Because green smoothies foster an alkaline environment, they are an excellent way to boost your immune system. I whip up green smoothies in my Vitamixer almost daily for a healthy meal on the go.

Generally, I have a sweet smoothie for breakfast and savory ones in the afternoon or evening. I tend to use whatever is in my kitchen, rather than following a recipe, although I have written up a few of my favorites for you here. For sweet smoothies, I usually include 2 fruits, 1 or 2 cups of greens, 1½ cups of water, and some superfoods (see below). My favorite fruits include all kinds of berries, bananas, mango, fresh figs, papaya, apples, pears, and plums. If it works with the mix, I'll use fresh lemon or lime juice and I like adding fresh spearmint to my morning smoothies when it is warmer, and fresh ginger if it's a cold morning. If I need something more filling, I may add half an avocado or some almonds to the mix.

For greens, my favorite is kale, then spinach, and chard. For those who find blended greens too bitter, add agave nectar to sweeten up your drink. I'm a sucker for the taste and consistency of coconut nectar, a juice blend, so I often add this if fresh coconut water isn't available. Regularly rotating the ingredients ensures optimal nourishment.

My savory smoothies almost always have a base of tomato, carrot, and greens, to which I add whatever other delicious items I have in the house along with a cup of water. Wonderful additions include cucumber, garlic cloves, avocado, parsley, cilantro, celery, sage, fresh lemon and/or lime, sprouts, apples, papaya, dulse, and basil. Sometimes when I'm feeling adventurous, I'll throw in some cayenne pepper and/or Tabasco, or Braggs Liquid Aminos for a nice zing!

I use superfoods to build stamina and boost my performance and endurance. They are rejuvenating substances that boost the immune system, increasing resistance to physical and emotional stress. The ones I highly recommend are: blue-green algae, spirulina, Dr. Greens Daily

Superfood, organic cracked cell chlorella, goji berries, flaxseed oil, raw coconut oil, and Peruvian Maca root powder. Two wonderful online resources for supplements and superfoods are www.sunfood.com and www.cafegratitude.com. Sometimes I use organic fresh bee pollen or royal jelly from a nearby source. When I need a protein boost, I'll use pea, hemp or whey protein, or cocoa nibs depending on my mood. I mix these superfoods right into the smoothies, but some, like Noni Juice and Gold Rush Colloidal Gold, I take alone as a single shot. Many of these superfoods contain vital enzymes, amino acids, and other micronutrients.

It feels really good to take time to nourish my body with radiant, glowing, live, raw foods. It shows in my hooping, my complexion, and my stamina. Plus, making smoothies is another form of creative expression: You can explore tastes and colors to delight your senses! Keep your kitchen stocked with seasonal produce and let your intuition guide you to try new combinations.

Here are some of my favorite recipes to get you started. Just toss all the ingredients into a food processor and blend until smooth. Careful not to overblend so they become frothy. Drink smoothies while fresh and store the remains in the refrigerator, where they'll keep for a day.

Sweet Smoothies

▶ RAINBOW TROPICAL DELIGHT

I love starting my day with this very nurturing smoothie with a delicious aftertaste.

- ½ pint strawberries
- ½ banana
- ½ avocado
- 1 plum
- 1 handful kale
- 2 teaspoons Maca powder
- 1 teaspoon bee pollen
- 1 tablespoon agave nectar
- 1 cup water

▶ GREEN SUNSHINE

This one's perfect for jump-starting a cloudy day.

- 1 bag prewashed spinach
- ½ basket fresh figs
- 1 apple, cored
- ⅓ bundle fresh spearmint leaves
- Barley grass powder
- 1 cup water

▶ COCONUT FANTASY

A tropical delight makes a great vacation after working the hoop!

- 7 leaves romaine lettuce
- 1 cup coconut nectar or ½ cup coconut water
- 2 dates
- 1 banana
- ½ fresh pineapple (peeled, cored, and cut in chunks)
- 1 cup water

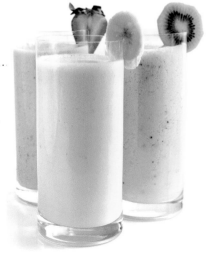

Savory Smoothies

▶ PELE'S POTION

Named after Pele, the Hawaiian goddess of volcanoes, fire, and dance, this smoothie will warm your core.

- 2 handfuls spinach
- 1 knob fresh ginger (peeled)
- Splash of Braggs Amino Acids
- ½ avocado
- 1 clove garlic

- ½ apple, seeded
- 1 carrot
- 1 large tomato (I love heirloom)
- ⅓ bunch cilantro
- ⅓ bunch parsley

- 1 tablespoon flaxseed oil
- Generous sprinkle cayenne pepper (optional)
- 1½ cups water

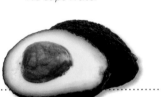

▶ SHAKA ZULU

Welcome spicy jungle power into your day with this recipe.

- ¾ bunch collard greens
- 1 tomato
- ¼ onion
- Handful fresh cilantro
- 1 clove minced garlic

- 1 knob fresh ginger (peeled)
- 1 stick celery
- ½ cucumber
- ½ avocado

- Juice from one lime, fresh squeezed
- Pinch cayenne (optional, and to taste)
- 1 cup water

▶ HEALING GARDEN

Herbs are amazing! Let them work their magic in your body.

- A couple of sprigs fresh sage
- A couple of sprigs fresh rosemary
- A couple of sprigs fresh thyme

- A couple of sprigs fresh parsley
- ½ avocado
- 1 apple (cored)
- Juice from ½ lemon

- 1 bag prewashed spinach
- 1 cup water

INDEX OF MOVES